Restack: A New Approach to Dismantle the Blocks Holding You Back

Do you have mental blocks keeping you from your goals? Have you tried multiple times to eat healthier, exercise more, decrease your stress, and get restful sleep, but the behavioral changes didn't stick? *Restack* is a book that embraces our humanness, with our quirks and imperfections, and provides tools and practical suggestions to *Restack* ourselves in a way that's psychologically freeing.

To *Restack* is the process of identifying our mental blocks and then categorizing and tweaking parts of ourselves we want to keep, as well as what is no longer serving us. The aim is not to create an idealized version of a perfect human, but to *Restack* the metaphorical tower of our blocks to end up with a new and reinvigorated *Restack* of ourselves.

Restack explores lifestyle interventions, backed by science, to propel us forward on our journey of both mental and physical health. The concepts presented are a part of the big puzzle of brain health—each piece of the puzzle affects our overall physical and emotional health, and how we can manage this impact through lifestyle interventions. The book contains multiple tables and figures, as well as "self-help prescriptions," all serving as tools to provide guidance and help you achieve your goals. Additionally, Gia Merlo, as a practicing psychiatrist, shares her journey through her imperfections, mistakes, and mental blocks to come to a place of self-acceptance and healing.

The ultimate goal of this book is not to be 100% healthy or 100% perfect, but to feel 100% *human* — actualizing our full human potential.

Advance Praise for *Restack*

"*Restack* by Dr. Gia Merlo offers a compelling blend of vulnerability and expertise, weaving personal narratives with professional insights in psychiatry and lifestyle medicine. The book's fresh approach and emphasis on self-compassion provides a valuable roadmap for those looking to navigate mental blocks and embark on a journey of self-discovery."

> – Wendy Suzuki, PhD, author of *Healthy Brain: Happy Life* and *Good Anxiety*, Professor of Neural Science and Dean of the of College of Arts and Science, New York University

"In this deeply personal and moving book, Dr. Merlo shares her innermost thoughts about her journey toward improved mental well-being, allowing the cracks and crevices of pain to show, but also sharing ways to heal. This is a must-read."

> – Uma Naidoo, MD, nutritional psychiatrist, Harvard Medical School, Chef, Culinary Instructor, author of *This is Your Brain on Food* and *Calm Your Mind with Food*

"*Restack* is a compelling exploration of self-discovery and transformation. Dr. Gia Merlo offers a rare and intimate glimpse into the human psyche, expertly guiding readers through the process of dismantling the barriers that impede our growth. This book is a testament to the resilience of the human spirit, providing a clear roadmap for anyone seeking to harness their full potential. A must-read for those ready to embark on a journey of healing, self-acceptance, and profound change."

> – Chef AJ, Chef AJ LIVE!

"This extraordinary book showcases Dr. Merlo's rare gift for vulnerability and authenticity, offering readers a deeply introspective and multifaceted exploration of the self. She uses her own experiences as a beacon of hope, making this book an indispensable companion on the journey of healing and self-development."

– Ali Saad, MD, neurologist, University of Colorado Anschutz Medical Campus

"*Restack* by Dr. Gia Merlo is a very brave book. Dr. Merlo is one of the most influential physicians in the world blending psychiatry and mental health with lifestyle medicine. She has made substantial contributions to both. The current book explores her own triumphs and heartbreaks and shares her deeply personal vulnerabilities. She combines this with authoritative information about psychiatry and mental health as well as lifestyle medicine. I hope this book gives other people the courage to look honestly at the ups and downs that all of us experience in our lives. As Rafiki in the Lion King admonished Simba 'The past can hurt. But you can either run from it or learn from it.' Dr. Merlo has shown us how to take our past and learn from it. It is an important message that is destined to help everyone who reads this insightful book."

– James Rippe, MD, cardiologist, author of 53 books, Editor-in-Chief, American Journal of Lifestyle Medicine and the Journal of Intensive Care Medicine

"What does it mean to be an innovator? How does someone know if something is innovative? Only history can answer these questions definitively, but don't be surprised when history confirms the creative impact of Dr. Gia Merlo on the field of psychiatry. *Restack* is an innovative, creative, fresh take on maximizing human potential through lifestyle modification. She offers a vulnerable, compelling narrative that is relatable to all people."

– Steve Sugden, MD MPH, psychiatrist, University of Utah Spencer Fox Eccles School of Medicine

"Dr. Gia Merlo is a courageous clinician, daring to disrupt the system. Her book is both powerful and moving!"
   – Beth Frates, MD, Harvard Medical School; President, American College of Lifestyle Medicine

"The book is truly **special** and valuable, not just fully packed by science, but also filled with heartfelt healing and connectedness from the personal stories that the author experienced and shared of basic human struggles, pains, fears, or burnouts that all human beings generally face in their life course. She is a renowned world leader in the field of Lifestyle Psychiatry. She stacks the remedies and roadmaps to help readers in this magical book.
   – Dr. Jenny Sunghyun Lee, The Founding Chair & CEO, Korean College of Lifestyle Medicine

"In *Restack*, we're invited to view mental blocks as the beginning of building blocks and to recognize that there is no perfect endpoint – rather, there can be a lifelong journey of learning and growth. Dr. Merlo deftly weaves the narrative of her own life, including traumas and disappointments, with real-world challenges we all face. She invites self-reflection, application of evidence-based lifestyle medicine strategies, and the cultivation of a learning approach to growth and change. Throughout, we're reminded that mental health and physical health are not separate and distinct – they are facets of our humanity and represent all that we can be!"
   – Simon Matthew, CEO, Wellcoaches® Australia and Wellcoaches® Singapore

"A huge THANK YOU to Dr. Gia Merlo—both for her incredible curiosity, scientific exploration and personal resilience; and for creating such an inspiring and practical roadmap for others to utilize during their own journey of health and healing. This book speaks to our craving to feel at home and content within our own bodies and minds. It encourages us **not** to strive to be 100% perfect—but, as Dr. Merlo explains, to be 100% human. Reading it feels like going for a walk while having a long conversation with a trusted friend and mentor. It provides the space for envisioning a new path and a more nurturing paradigm, one *Restack* at a time."

> – Meagan L. Grega, MD, FACLM, Chief Medical Officer, *Kellyn Foundation*

"We live and work in increasingly complex and dynamic times. Much is expected of us all both in our personal and professional lives. And often we are our loudest and strongest critics holding us back from being our best selves. *Restack* provides a roadmap for leading a happier and more successful life. A compelling and timely read."

> – Patricia Davidson, PhD, Vice-Chancellor and President, University of Wollongong, Australia

"*Restack* is an honest and compassionate gift of Dr. Gia Merlo, whose wisdom and experiences will surely offer both consolation and healing to those seeking wholeness. Dr. Merlo's personal and professional identities are beautifully interwoven, bringing stories together with evidence-based science, and centering the narrative that lifestyle strategies are key building blocks of health and fulfillment."

> – Lianna Levine Reisner, Network Director, Plant Powered Metro New York

"In this book, Dr. Gia Merlo courageously shares her personal story as well as insights from her work as a psychiatrist and lifestyle medicine physician. She lays out how we can uncover our personal truths and embrace our situation with self-compassion in order to boost our wellbeing. Getting unstuck and moving forward in a positive direction requires that we reframe our lifestyle approach authentically. Through engaging and relatable stories, *Restack* lays out why and how we can progress to becoming our best selves."

> – Liana Lianov, MD, MPH, President, Global Positive Health Institute

"In this remarkable book, Dr. Merlo invites readers to embark on a journey of personal growth and actualization, drawing inspiration from her own narrative and fortified by decades of practicing psychotherapy and lifestyle medicine. This book is sure to inspire."

> – Douglas Noordsy, MD, psychiatrist, Stanford University School of Medicine

"As Dr. Merlo notes, this book truly is the culmination of her life's academic and personal work. Having worked with Dr. Merlo for the past decade, I can attest that she has walked-the-walk with the information presented in this book. Her knowledge and expertise in psychiatry, health care professionalism, and as a pioneer in lifestyle medicine and psychiatry, is incredible. That she has now taken her knowledge and her lived experiences to create an effective roadmap for others toward better mental and physical health is a gift."

> – Thomas Harter, PhD, Director of Bioethics, Gundersen Health System

Restack

A New Approach to Dismantle
the Blocks Holding You Back

Gia Merlo, MD

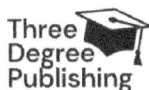

Three
Degree
Publishing

Treatment for conditions described in this material is highly dependent on the individual circumstances. No book can replace the diagnostic expertise and medical advice of a trusted physician. Please consult with your doctor before making any decisions that affect your health, especially if you suffer from any medical symptoms or conditions that require treatment. The information or guidance contained within this book are provided simply as a supplement to a medical professional's judgment on appropriate treatments. This book does not indicate whether a treatment is suited for a particular person. Because of the rapid advances of medical science, any information, recommendations, diagnoses, and Rx's should be independently verified. The publisher and the author make no representations or warranties as to the accuracy or efficacy of the mentioned information. The authors and the publisher do not accept, and expressly disclaim, any responsibility for any liability, loss, or risk that may be claimed or incurred as a consequence of the use and/or application of any of the contents of this material. The content of this book and the views contained within are the opinions of the author and not of any affiliated institutions. Any references to patients and cases are not actual patients but a fictitious representation and any likeness to actual people is a coincidence and accidental.

for Torin

Though just a toddler
he is teaching us all
how to *Restack* blocks
with intention, joy, and laughter

Table of Contents (Overview)

Tables

Figures

Rx's

Table of Contents (Detailed)

About Gia Merlo, MD, MBA, MEd

Dr. Gia Merlo is a clinical professor of psychiatry and nursing at New York University and NYU Grossman School of Medicine, associate editor of the American Journal of Lifestyle Medicine, founding chair of the Lifestyle Psychiatry Caucus of the American Psychiatric Association, and a fellow of the American College of Lifestyle Medicine. She is a part of the Faculty Group Practice at NYU Langone Health in New York City. She completed her Master of Education in Health Professions at Johns Hopkins University School of Education in August 2022 and is currently an Adjunct Faculty at Johns Hopkins helping students in the program complete their capstone projects. She has published numerous peer-reviewed articles, chapters in books, and published four academic books for healthcare professionals with Oxford University Press and Taylor and Francis.

Merlo has been curious about and interested in lifestyle interventions, especially concerning the overlap of mental and physical health. She is thrilled to write a self-help book that is firmly grounded in science. In this book, the science is drawn from psychology, psychiatry, and lifestyle medicine and her personal narratives are sprinkled throughout in an accessible and helpful way.

In her spare time, Dr. Merlo enjoys playing tennis, not taking herself too seriously as she re-learns how to play violin (after many, many years) in a community orchestra, and hiking in New York and New Jersey. She finds great joy watching a good comedy that allows her to fulfill her daily health prescription dose of laughing out loud.

Connect via giamerlo.com and linkedin.com/in/giamerlomd, @DrGiaMerlo, and https://www.instagram.com/giamerlomd/

Introduction

I have made many mistakes in my life. Over the years I've often seen myself get healthier and then fall back to square one—over-analyzing the roads I took and continuously grappling with the choices that affect who I am, who I was and ultimately who I will become.

My journey in medical school began at the age of 18, fresh-faced and straight out of high school. I got married and had a child shortly thereafter. Navigating medical school and residency became more difficult after my divorce, as my daughter was still an infant. Very little support was available to a woman working as both a physician and as the sole provider for her child in the 1990s. I found it challenging and exhausting to shift between taking care of my patients, being a mother, and compartmentalizing the pain and suffering from my sexually, physically, and emotionally abusive marriage.

Working to overcome these traumas over the next few decades informed my continued growth as a psychiatrist. Over my 30-year career, I have engaged in numerous rounds of psychotherapy and dabbled in self-help. Teasing out my role and responsibility in the ups and downs of my life has not been easy. However, the process has helped me connect and empathize with my patients and understand the quiet suffering of others.

Writing this book has been a departure from what my career has been focused on thus far. After I finished my residency, I spent 40 to 60 hours each week seeing patients, with little to no time for much else. During the past few years, I have pivoted to writing academic books and journal articles, which, if I were lucky, would be read by other health professionals. And if they were read, it would take 5, 10, or often 15 years for the concepts to trickle down and impact the lives of the community. *Restack* shares what I've learned from my life, my patients, my students, my family, my blunders, and ultimately my joys to a wider audience— you.

The process of organizing and drafting *Restack* has stirred a whirlwind of emotions within me. Crafting my personal journey into a series of words on a page and sharing these intimate details has required me to dismantle pieces of myself, take a hard look at what I've done, how I feel about it, and face what has held me back. I've found myself embarrassed more times than you can imagine. I ask myself constantly: Is my story worth it? Will anybody want to read it? And more importantly, will my vulnerability inspire readers to better themselves—or will they dismiss it and pass judgment on me?

I experienced numerous profound realizations in my own psychotherapy over the years, which left me feeling better and closer to where I wanted to be, but still not quite there. For example, if I treated one of my issues, such as addressing my role in the abuse within my marriage, this healing of one aspect of myself would cause misalignment in others. I would be left with raw, unresolved experiences and emotions. The imbalances were unsettling at best, and disruptive at worst. Yet, I went through this alignment-misalignment hundreds of times as I worked on myself, refusing to allow the setbacks to derail me, and learning more about myself with each round.

But, how does this process relate to this book?

Tower of Blocks

Let's use the analogy of a tower of blocks that a child might build. If we visualize individual aspects of ourselves as the blocks that make up the tower, we recognize that some of them are structural and serve to hold the tower up, while some can be easily removed without the tower falling. In psychotherapy, it can be unclear how crucial the piece of us we're working on is to our foundation. In other words, by addressing one aspect of ourselves that we want to change, we might inadvertently disrupt the balance of the tower, necessitating a process of realignment.

In other cases, we may want to "remove" some blocks, such as our explosive angry selves, and say "good riddance." Or we may use compassion and kindness to work on other parts, for example, any part of ourselves that was mistreated. We also may want to strengthen and solidify other blocks to become a part of our foundation, such as the ability to love ourselves and form mutually supportive relationships.

Blocks versus Mental Blocks

I also want to differentiate the two terms: (1) building blocks of the tower and (2) *mental blocks*. In this book, I play off both uses of the word *block*.

As we established before, some building blocks may be necessary for the integrity of the structure, and some can be easily removed. If we view some blocks as potentially healthy, and others as unhealthy, then we can make the leap into the analogy of our mental blocks.

Mental blocks can be multifaceted—not as simple as they appear on the surface. We may want to remove some mental blocks entirely, some we may gently adjust to get to where we want to be, and some we may want to live with. For example, someone might be content with their overly cerebral point-of-view because it helps them excel at their job, whereas another person might struggle with constantly being "in their head," particularly if they feel like it interferes with their personal relationships. Not everyone is the same. It's about what *you* want, how you envision *your* full potential.

What Is Restack?

Restack-ing is the process of identifying the pieces, deciding what we want to keep, replacing what does not work, adjusting our infrastructure, and ending up with a new and reinvigorated *Restack* of what we like. To reiterate, the goal of *Restack*-ing is not always to change everything in all parts of ourselves. Our aim is not to create an idealized version of a "perfect human." Even the unhealthy parts of ourselves serve a purpose within our whole. That's why it is often so hard to change our deeper psychological issues. The deeper the issues, the more intricately woven they are into the core structure of who we are. In this analogy, the deepest issues may be the most foundational for the tower.

For example, if we engage in psychotherapy, we are often encouraged to view our lived experiences and internal psyche through a different lens. An internal change in perspective is often necessary to reframe an experience; a perceived failure can frequently be an opportunity for growth. When we do this, we sometimes dredge up mental blocks that then need to be reprocessed and framed in a healthier way. Please note, as we are working to change ourselves, there are multiple points where a restack may be warranted. In Chapter 9 the *Restack Model of Change* is proposed as a fresh way of addressing the content here within.

We are all constantly *Restack*-ing, whether we know it or not. This book helps us through that process.

The Evolution of *Restack*

So, why did I write this book? I believe my own psychotherapy treatment, my work in the mental health field, academic book writing and editing, and personal self-help have all been valuable elements of my journey. I wanted this book to integrate and bring all these elements together. My hope is that you can learn from what has and what hasn't worked for me. Maybe you will find this conversation useful.

Sitting down to draft this book has been complex. It has taken me four attempts. Not four revisions, but I have written four different unpublished books to get to this one.

The first version was started with my student, Ariyaneh Nikbin, as she transcribed an 80,000-word autobiographical text of my life journey that was full of the retelling of multiple intense traumas from my marriage. I gained some healing from writing the narrative and having a bright, evolved person to share the experience with. Looking back on it, I realize I was exploring the reparative powers of narrative writing. But how many people would want to read someone's raw pain and traumatic experiences without a consolidation and synthesis of the information, and some inspirational message? I know that version could have been triggering for many readers and could be experienced as *trauma dumping*. Thus, the project was abandoned.

My second endeavor was more of an educational book, focusing on aspects of our human experience, without sharing much of my story. Ultimately, that message didn't feel like the one I wanted to share. It was detached and didn't include my voice. It didn't feel authentic.

For my third attempt, I wrote a 15-chapter book, with each chapter highlighting a patient I had treated. It included therapy dialogues, with the hope of identifying common *aha* moments during the process of psychotherapy. Though a useful approach, that draft also did not resonate with my ultimate goal. I don't want anyone to think I have all the answers, or that I'm a perfect human therapizing others while having no issues of my own. Indeed, I am a lifelong learner and lifelong *Restack*-er.

So, *Restack* is my fourth attempt. And hopefully, the processes I went through in the previous three versions helped solidify the lessons I present in this book, as well as my journey. Within the lifestyle medicine movement, many clinicians share their stories of improvement in their chronic *physical* diseases, such as heart or autoimmune diseases, with lifestyle interventions. Practicing clinicians sharing their *mental* health journeys are rare and even more so in the lifestyle medicine movement. I hope this book helps bridge that gap and opens the floor for more conversations and transparency. The time has come for all of us to share our humanness—it helps our patients, and it helps us.

My Journey

I have had a nagging feeling something was missing numerous times in my life.

I have experienced much shame and pain in not being able to address some very real and obvious mental blocks. I went through a period where I was in different romantic relationships, all of which taught me a lot. However, I was in my 40s then, and I often thought that these growth periods ought to have happened while I was a younger person. My lack of experience and perceived disconnection from other adults my age frustrated me. I was uncomfortable with many aspects of myself, including my emotional eating. After all, I was a physician—in fact, a psychiatrist—and able to help others work through their difficult relationships with food. Why couldn't I help myself? What were my mental blocks, and how could I address them?

The reality was, even though I had healed parts of my past trauma, I was still struggling with my weight. Over time, I realized I was padding myself, meaning I was putting on extra weight to make myself feel less attractive. I had no idea if others found me less attractive, but this tactic gave me an excuse to not date. It was my internal way of avoiding intimacy and, therefore, protecting myself from being hurt again after my traumatic marriage.

My lack of confidence was such that not only did I not date, but I also didn't feel adequate as a parent for my child. I thought she needed to spend time with relatives because they could provide something I lacked. To be sure, my daughter having a relationship with her extended family was good for her. I'm not questioning that. My motivation for the interaction, however, was ill-conceived. Was my lack of confidence in my parenting ultimately playing out in the family in unhealthy ways? It's taken me a long time to realize what I had, who I was, and *who I am* are more than enough. The mental blocks that prevented me from feeling confident required a *Restack*.

It's genuinely heartwarming now to witness my adult daughter and her husband interact with their young son. They laugh with such abandon as he curiously and confidently absorbs his surroundings. The love and comfort my grandson receives is delightful to see. Children don't need two parents. They don't even need one perfect parent. Our partners don't need us to be perfect either. As humans, we need trust and unconditional love. Everything else is a bonus.

My aim in this book is to share what I've learned so at least one person will feel heard and not shy away or slow down on their journey to live a life with their full human potential. I hope each person who reads this book can understand that who they *are* and what they *have* is enough.

Part A: The Foundation

Chapter 1: Why Read This Book?

Everyone Googles.

Clearly, we have tons of information available to us on the Internet. We know we need to eat healthfully, exercise, and get enough sleep. The goal of these behaviors is to have the fullest human experience with the best quality of life—to feel good, have energy, and be in good health.

We all have an abundance of lived experiences that interplay with our genetic predispositions and intergenerational values. We are constantly integrating these experiences into who we are and who we become. We are ever-changing—that is the basis of being human. Each of us has a different path in this integration of lived experiences. We end up with a complex inner world of emotions, feelings, thoughts, and personalities unique to each one of us.

These interacting elements of our experience can either impede us from reaching our human potential or be *Restack*-ed on our journey to becoming the best version of ourselves. To *Restack*, we must first take an inventory of what makes us human, such as our traumas, emotions, thoughts, and personality traits. We must also look at the external environment, such as our work and social determinants of health, which also interact with our internal human qualities. The goal is to tweak what we can—reshuffle, reorganize, realign, refine, and revitalize these elements.

We will never be perfect. But we will always be 100% human. Part of our humanness is our quirks and imperfections. Finding a way to *Restack* obstacles and unhelpful habits may free us up to move toward our full human potential. Wouldn't that be a fabulous end goal in our growth?

Questions We Take for Granted

From childhood to adulthood, we grow and evolve in many different dimensions. As adults, we find ourselves stuck with desirable and undesirable traits and habits we have developed over our lifetime. Because we are part of a society, we take many societal standards as norms. On a personal level, it's also easy to stick with our status quo and become stagnant.

With our plates already full of daily responsibilities, who has the time to question these norms, find answers, and take action? But answering such questions is necessary for us to continue to evolve.

Questions like:
Why do we eat what we eat, and why are we unable to change our habits even when we know it is harmful?
Why do we continue to smoke when we know it causes cancer?

And some of these are deeper and existential questions:
Why do we measure success the way we do?
Has "success" brought fulfillment into our lives?
Why am I always lonely?

Others address the ingrained norms in society we have often accepted as truth, such as:
Why do we have a five-day workweek?
Why do schools run from 9 am to 3 pm when most families have two working parents?
Why do we think a certain body physique is more attractive than another (history has shown that wasn't always so)?
Why did 10,000 steps a day become the standard for daily steps needed for health?

Because these questions are often uninvestigated and unanswered, we may develop barriers in these areas of our lives that prevent us from achieving what we want. Some of us will externalize the pressure of knowing the truth and hold on tightly to our internal biases. Others of us will see these patterns repeat again and again and be compelled to dig deeply within ourselves to understand the causes and disrupt the cycles.

What can we do to dispel these unexamined societal norms so that we can continue in our personal growth?

This book hopes to address that. Before delving in, let's first look at the structure of this book.

Prescriptions, Tables, and Figures

Often abbreviated as Rx, a *prescription* is defined as a recommended treatment to help alleviate disease or suffering. Our society has evolved to view medications as the only treatment form that goes on a prescription. The Rx pad, historically, has been used for this singular purpose. Now, physicians' Rx pads are almost exclusively electronic, furthering the narrow definition of an Rx. Indeed, these electronic communications go straight to pharmacists who dispense the prescribed treatments, reinforcing the common notion that treatments are necessarily medications.

In this book, I am expanding the use of Rx's ("Rx's" is an acceptable plural form of Rx in the medical literature) to include other interventions that, while not being medication-based, also alleviate suffering and promote a healthy lifestyle. These would be in the form of reflections, thought exercises, activities, and assessments. While all the Rx's in this book may not resonate with or be the right treatments for everyone, they are meant as guidance and tools for your self-help journey. Where appropriate, I also include tables and figures to help clarify and consolidate the information presented in the text.

Cases Used in the Book

Throughout the book, multiple cases from my clinical experience as a psychiatrist are presented to highlight the concepts in the chapters. In the case presentations, I incorporate evidence-based solutions I have learned and discovered through my work. Please note the patient case reports have all been de-identified and altered to protect my patients' privacy. In addition, I use my personal narrative to share my mistakes, biases, and struggles. While I removed most of the harrowing details in the cases to minimize potential triggers, please forgive me for any narrative that may be difficult to read.

As a psychiatrist focused on clinical work, authoring this book has been an evolution in my own understanding of how to help people. Many of us may feel that we could benefit from altering parts of ourselves here and there, and I have been very successful in reshaping parts of myself over the years. No one reading this book has asked me to perform an evaluation of them, and I don't know each reader and their particular circumstance on an individual basis. Therefore, I don't have the knowledge to guide you individually. But, I do have about 30 years of clinical experience in gently guiding others and myself. Some tweaks have been easier than others. Believe me, I've made a lot of mistakes and facing them hasn't always been easy. Oftentimes, it's a case of two steps forward, one step back.

You might ask why I give examples of my personal evolution through the good, bad, and ugly of my lived experiences? I have recounted them here to help remove the shame surrounding the discussion of mental and emotional hardships, and to bring to the forefront of the conversation some topics that are often difficult to deal with, including death, dying, and trauma.

Parts of This Book

I have organized this book into four parts to guide us as we embark on our journey of *Restack*-ing, going from mental blocks to our full human potential. The four parts are (A) The Foundation, (B) Mental Blocks, (C) External Barriers, and (D) Solutions for Everyone. As a bonus, I end the book with an epilogue where I try to pull together my journey for the reader.

Part A

Part A, The Foundation, consists of Chapters 1 and 2 where I introduce how we can improve our mental health and even treat mental illness by using lifestyle interventions to make incremental changes in our brains. The material in Chapter 2 is dense, but please bear with me. I feel it's important to educate ourselves about lifestyle psychiatry and brain health, so we understand we have the power to alter the way our brain functions. This can, in turn, facilitate lasting adjustments in our behaviors. Our psychological habits, such as spending hours scrolling on our phones or worrying excessively about something we said are not elusive behaviors to which we have no access—brain science shows these habits can often be understood and intervened upon.

Part B

Part B, Mental Blocks, consists of Chapters 3 through 6. In this book, the mental blocks include the pieces of ourselves that may obstruct our growth or progress. These pieces may start externally as trauma but can ultimately cause psychological and physiological changes within us. Therefore, Chapter 3 is titled "Internalized Trauma." Other chapters in this part discuss our emotion regulation, cognitive states, and personality traits. Many of us struggle with obstacles that prevent us from achieving our full potential, even when we know exactly what we need to do.

Self-help books, by nature, introduce tools and describe methods we can use to change our habits. Often these books start the conversation with an assumption that changing habits will change a process that happens inside of us. For many of us, addressing the habits we don't like may lead to permanent and positive changes in our lives. But some of us may be left frustrated and confused and no closer to our goal. We may read these books, employ the tools presented, and when no change occurs, feel like we're a failure. Or we may wonder if we did something wrong because we're continuing to exhibit behaviors we so desperately want to change. In my opinion, addressing the mental blocks presented in Chapters 3-6 is key to creating long-lasting changes for most of us.

Part C

Part C, External Barriers, consists of Chapters 7 and 8. After addressing the foundations of brain health and our mental blocks in Parts A and B, we move onto a vital area of discussion that is often overlooked. The external barriers addressed in this book are complex and varied. I delve into the nature of our working lives, including burnout, and social determinants of health. While many of us use the term "burnout" to also include non-work-related stressors, this chapter may not be as relevant, but instead Chapter 13 on "Stress Management" addresses non-work related burnout more effectively. Some external barriers, if severe enough or present for long enough, may become internalized and lead to internal blocks. For example, in the medical literature, burnout is a term associated with chronic work-related stress. But over time, burnout may lead to emotional dysregulation, negative self-talk, and changes in our personality traits, such as becoming overly critical. Though I treat these external barriers chapters separately, the concepts are deeply intertwined with the content laid out in the rest of the book. Then in Chapter 8, environmental factors, such as air quality and the heat index, are explored.

Part D

Part D starts out in Chapter 9 discussing behavioral change and my *Restack Model of Change.* Multiple Rx's describe the steps in getting ready to change, goal setting, and ultimately sustaining change. Chapters 10 through 17 empowers us to seek solutions by employing lifestyle interventions with restorative sleep, physical activity and movement, nutrition, stress reduction, relationships (to ourselves, others and the world-at-large), and substance use harm reduction. Society has decided for us through advertising and social templates what is healthy and not healthy, and we generally believe and internalize this information, whether it's accurate or not. The misinformation we absorb can be categorized as intentional (which can be a form of manipulation) or unintentional (which may be well-meaning). I have to believe most of the misinformation we receive about lifestyle health is unintentional. In Part D, I hope to distill the research data and empower you, the reader, with the healthiest lifestyle interventions for the blocks you can recognize. The aim is to help us get back on the health trajectory that was our innate goal before we were derailed by our acquired mental blocks. Ultimately, my desire is that we fully embrace living life with joy, health, and happiness.

The Overarching Goal

Let's not strive to be 100% healthy or 100% perfect but instead to be *100% human.*

The goal of the interventions, whether we're talking about the mental blocks of Part B or the lifestyle interventions of Part D, is not to achieve a perfect bill of health or a perfect lifestyle. It does mean being able to return to the trajectory we would have taken if we hadn't been burdened with certain lived experiences or external barriers influencing our mental health.

Lived experiences make us who we are. Of course, we don't want to be living in George Orwell's *1984* with each of us losing our individuality, but we want to be free of the weight of the internalized consequences of our negative lived experiences for our health and our planet.

Not Only Personal Health, but Also Planetary Health

There is no point in being human and feeling *100% human* if we don't have a planet to live on. As we go through the process of *Restack*-ing for our personal mental and physical health, I would argue we need to consider how societal norms have affected the planet's health.

What we eat is something we take for granted. Yet we spend an inordinate amount of time and energy depleting the planet of important nutrients by overgrazing and producing gasses, which affect our environment. We have enough food in the food production system to feed every one of us in this world. The water and feed required to harvest animals for human consumption could be instead used to feed families directly.[1] We must stop and take a hard look at our practices if we plan to survive on this planet. The health implications of the way we live for our bodies are huge for our bodies, but even more importantly, the health of our planet is at stake. This is discussed in more detail in Chapter 8: Our Environment and Health.

Humans Are Not Meant to Be Perfect

Once we establish that perfection is a laudable goal, but not a natural state as humans, perhaps we can have more compassion, empathy, and forgiveness for ourselves when we are less than perfect. How many of us make mistakes, pause to reflect, get back up, and learn from them? And how many of us make mistakes, sit down and cringe, blame ourselves, and criticize ourselves for our humanness? I would argue that, as a species, we're too hard on ourselves. Our expectations have blended and overlapped between our professional need to be perfect and our genetic drive to be human.

Being the best version of ourselves, gentle, and self-compassionate is something those blessed with families who embrace diversity and individual differences in their children may consider automatic. Yet applying this to our personal and professional adult experiences often requires intention.

I have seen many people show compassion to their children in their personal lives, but then become harsh and unforgiving to themselves and those around them in their workplace. How does this dichotomy happen? The disconnect between how we envision responsibilities at work and in our personal lives is an interesting phenomenon to consider. Many times, we have a *fractionated internal schema* of what work is and what family is. Fractionated internal schema is a mental framework resulting in the compartmentalization of our work self and our home self, often because we function as a different person in each of these two settings. Internally, we keep these versions of ourselves as separate, distinct identities without sharing the knowledge, emotions, and feelings between the two. In adulthood, we have control over the separate identities, and therefore maintain memory between the two and it's much less severe and just seen as "parts" of ourselves–our work self and our home self. Should we reconcile these two versions of ourselves to form a more seamless identity? Should we, for example, bring aspects of our humanness to work?

What this requires is making incremental change, as much as is manageable, without feeling overwhelmed. We naturally feel stress when we make changes, but too much stress can leave us feeling defeated, which is counterproductive and can undermine our progress. By making small pivots across a range of lifestyle factors, rather than trying to solve 100% of any one issue, we may see tangible progress.

The internalized fractionated schema, though could be experienced as problematic, is not a diagnosable medical condition. In contrast to when this happens in childhood, the condition is known as dissociative identity disorder, (formally known as multiple personality disorder or MPD), where control of the distinct identities occurs with memory lapses between them. If you or someone you know struggles with memory lapses between identities, please seek appropriate professional treatment, as discussed in Chapter 16.

Evidence-Based Research on Lifestyle

This book aims to bring disparate neurological and cognitive research into one place. As a psychiatrist working with adults and children, I have spent about 30 years working in a variety of settings, including academic, clinical, and research. Over the years, my professional work included scholarly activity around medical professionalism, lifestyle medicine, and medical education, while maintaining a private practice. I have written peer-reviewed publications and have published four academic textbooks. With *Restack*, I'm drawing heavily on the research presented in an academic textbook I published with Christopher P. Fagundes titled *Lifestyle Psychiatry: Through the Lens of Behavioral Medicine*.[2]

By making this research accessible to a general reader, I hope to facilitate self-help within the realm of lifestyle. Overall, numerous factors bar access to receiving care for mental health. We have a short supply of trained psychiatrists, clinical psychologists, and therapists, and the cost is often prohibitive for many people. If we can put the tools directly into the hands of individuals who need them, my hope is the impact of the research will land exactly where it is needed most. Indeed, I hope some readers will use this book as a resource on their journey to optimal health.

Who Should Read This Book?

Who would enjoy this book? This book is written for all readers who want to make changes within themselves to live the life they want, for those who have dabbled in self-help and therapy and still feel like something's still missing, and for those who have done everything to change their lifestyle behaviors but are not yet where they want to be.

As you read, please note that each chapter touches on how the concepts presented in the chapter are a part of the big puzzle of human brain health. In turn, we will examine how each piece of the puzzle affects our overall physical and emotional health, and how we can manage this impact through lifestyle interventions. Any one of these pieces of the puzzle can tip the scale in the direction of better health and improved functioning. In Chapter 14, we introduce the concept of *connectedness*. Connectedness includes social connection, an important topic to address while the epidemic of social isolation affects our health. Reaching beyond social connection, connectedness also includes our connection to ourselves, such as happiness, our meaning and purpose in life, in addition to our connection to the community at large, as with nature and spirituality. We will discuss how brain health can help build the body's resilience to both internal and external threats.

My hope is that, through reading this book, you will discover you can make changes within yourself to live the life you want. We can all address these barriers. But do we know what tools are needed and how to use them? This has been the story of my life, not knowing how to free myself up enough psychologically to live the life I want.

Perhaps you have been traumatized. Or do you have emotional or cognitive patterns interfering with your well-being? Are elements of your personality keeping you from your dreams? As a psychiatrist, I have studied these issues, not only for my patients, but also for myself. Indeed, facing my miscalculations, misjudgments, errors, and mistakes has afforded me a robust education. I can mostly look back and smile in understanding at my younger self as I continue my imperfect journey.

In *Restack*, I share these stories with you to let you know you are not alone, and you've got this! If I can do it, anyone can. With this book, I hope to instill in you the same passion and excitement I have for personal transformation. Ultimately, I want you to see this book as a tool to help you free yourself of the barriers stopping you from living the life you always wanted with joy.

Let's Address the Root Cause

Many of the most common diseases are lifestyle-related and can be traced back to an inflammatory process.

The framework we will be using is corroborated by research showing how many of these disease states, mental and physical, share common pathways of inflammation within the body. Addressing the root cause of the inflammatory process in our body can often reverse seemingly unrelated disease states (discussed more in Chapter 2). For example, a person's mood and arthritis symptoms may both improve together. In light of these discoveries, the way we have historically categorized diseased states may no longer be relevant and will need to be reoriented. A comprehensive discussion of specific disorders is beyond the scope of this book, but they are clearly presented in the sources I have cited and listed on my website www.giamerlo.com. I ask you to be patient as I build each of the pieces of my argument toward an eventual synthesis, and to have an open mind in considering an alternate way of approaching mental and physical health.

As I look to the future, I see a time when those of us who have struggled with multiple failed treatments will finally find relief. For example, veterans with previously treatment-resistant posttraumatic stress disorder (PTSD), those afflicted with egregious traumas, and patients who have struggled with severe depression for decades amid a poor quality of life will be able to bring their brains back to optimal functioning.

Just to be clear, for many of us, such lifestyle interventions are pieces of the puzzle that can't be effectively engaged with until we address the mental blocks I mentioned earlier. Once these obstacles are identified with the help of Part B, their resolutions will help determine which interventions may be the most effective for our particular journey to *100% human*.

For decades, people have entrusted me with their health, and I'm grateful for their trust and for all that I've learned from the journeys of my patients. As more data has become available, my own understanding has also evolved, and I endeavor to join the reader in continuing to evolve toward more useful, compassionate, and evidence-based approaches to our overall health. It's an exciting time in the field of health. Thank you for reading this book. I hope the way I've synthesized the information will be helpful to you, and I welcome conversation and feedback. Let's begin.

Chapter 2: Lifestyle Psychiatry and Brain Health

Where are the causes of mental illness located? The brain? The body? The soul? And how about physical illness? Are physical and mental illness connected? What is the science behind this? Let's explore these foundational questions.

Historical Context of Psychiatry

Historically, the science of psychiatry was questionable.

That led many people, especially those within the medical disciplines, to doubt those suffering from sadness, anxiety, or addictions really had an actual medical condition. Please note not all medical conditions need the same sort of treatment, and not all people suffering will respond to identical treatments the same way. It's a complex interaction. In this chapter, we delve into the science of mental health, which serves as a foundation for the rest of the book.

We've come a long way in the medical field of psychiatry—from the fifth century BCE when we believed people were demonically possessed, to Hippocrates who believed all mental illness has a biological cause (*the four humors*), to surgically removing parts of the brain in mentally ill patients in the 1800s. Over the next century, we moved from psychoanalysis being the solution for everyone to a 180-degree flip where everyone needed medication. While psychotherapy and/or medication can be very helpful for many of us, an all-or-nothing approach is not so helpful. Now, emerging science uses cutting-edge technology and its applications to better understand what happens when we are struggling with psychiatric symptoms.

This robust evolution of the medical field of psychiatry is robust and depicted in Figure 2.1. We have adapted to increasing knowledge and will continue to do so as more brain science becomes available. The use of artificial intelligence in psychiatry, psychedelics, digital mental health, precision medicine and lifestyle psychiatry are all in our conversations today and in the future transformation of the field.

Definition of Mental Health and Brain Health

What exactly does *mental health* mean? Is there an identified place in the body called "mental"?

All other specialties in medicine have a target organ. For example, cardiologists deal with the heart, nephrologists are kidney experts, and dermatologists focus on the skin. Do psychiatrists have an organ they treat? Many people would say no. By not having a target organ, psychiatry is often assumed to be or labeled as not a science or even a field of medicine.

But the organ psychiatrists are concerned with is the *brain*. Historically, the concept of brain health has been discussed as part of the expertise of neurologists and geriatric physicians treating Alzheimer's and other dementias. Through the previous centuries, the field of psychiatry has been unable to rely on laboratory and other scientific tests to diagnose psychiatric disorders. We're now arriving at a point where hard science is available, pushing the real brain changes observed in psychiatric disorders to the forefront. Using techniques such as functional magnetic resonance imaging (commonly abbreviated as fMRI), we can now visualize specific regions of the brain for many disorders, like depression and anxiety.[3,4,5,6,7] This exciting explosion of knowledge has the potential to prevent, slow, and sometimes reverse the symptoms as well as the root causes of many cognitive deficits and psychiatric disorders.

FIGURE 2.1 EVOLUTION OF THE MEDICAL FIELD OF PSYCHIATRY

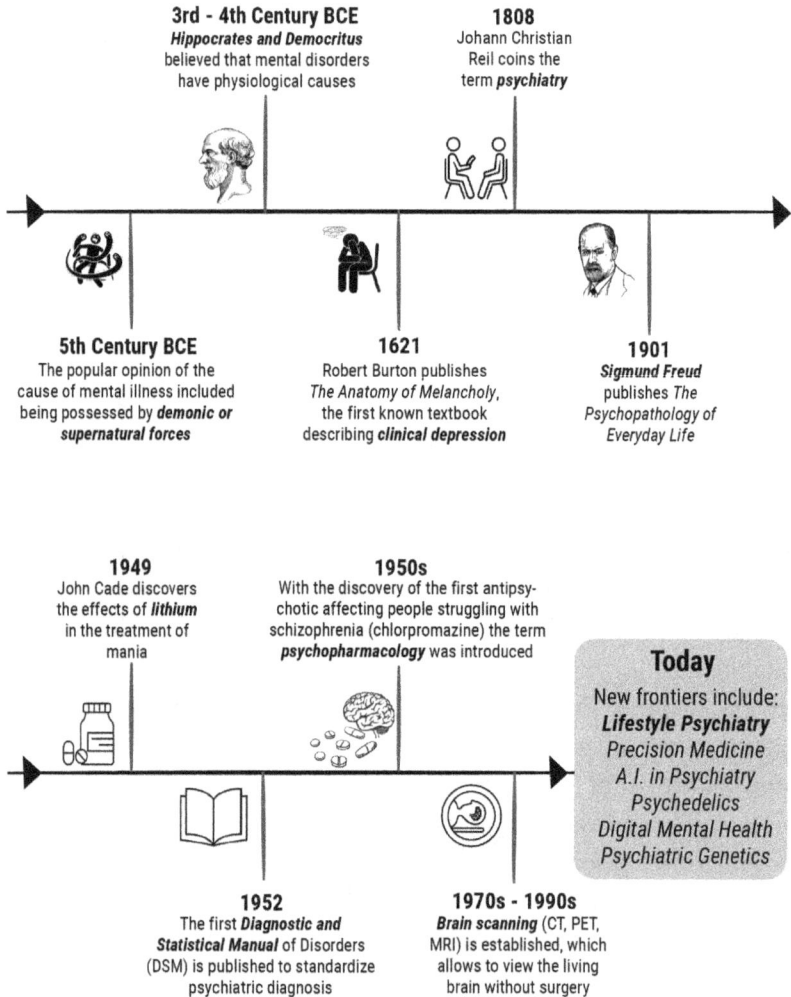

3rd - 4th Century BCE
Hippocrates and Democritus
believed that mental disorders
have physiological causes

1808
Johann Christian
Reil coins the
term *psychiatry*

5th Century BCE
The popular opinion of the
cause of mental illness included
being possessed by *demonic or
supernatural forces*

1621
Robert Burton publishes
The Anatomy of Melancholy,
the first known textbook
describing *clinical depression*

1901
Sigmund Freud
publishes *The
Psychopathology of
Everyday Life*

1949
John Cade discovers
the effects of *lithium*
in the treatment of
mania

1950s
With the discovery of the first antipsy-
chotic affecting people struggling with
schizophrenia (chlorpromazine) the term
psychopharmacology was introduced

Today
New frontiers include:
Lifestyle Psychiatry
Precision Medicine
A.I. in Psychiatry
Psychedelics
Digital Mental Health
Psychiatric Genetics

1952
The first *Diagnostic and
Statistical Manual* of Disorders
(DSM) is published to standardize
psychiatric diagnosis

1970s - 1990s
Brain scanning (CT, PET,
MRI) is established, which
allows to view the living
brain without surgery

Lifestyle Psychiatry

Lifestyle psychiatry is an emerging field in healthcare targeting interventions for psychological, social, and behavioral changes for optimal health and well-being.[2] Thousands of board-certified physicians now practice under the broader discipline, called lifestyle medicine, which has been gaining traction for the last few decades. Lifestyle medicine applies lifestyle interventions as a primary modality to prevent, treat, and often reverse chronic diseases, such as diabetes, heart disease, and obesity.

The field of lifestyle psychiatry also encompasses wellness, well-being, and lifestyle interventions for mental and brain health. We define wellness as a state of positive health that includes a person's quality of life and sense of well-being. Well-being, consequently, is how people feel and function with others and by themselves. Mental health encompasses wellness and well-being, in addition to the freedom from symptoms of mental illness. Brain health, in turn, embodies mental health as well as cognitive health across the lifespan.[8,9] In time, I hope we will be able to pivot and say all psychiatrists are "brain health doctors." But for now, we are commonly relegated to being "mental health doctors." Within this book, I will use the term *mental health* for psychiatric conditions as it is the most commonly used term at this time.

I'm often asked about the difference between interventions for someone who doesn't have a psychiatric diagnosis and someone who does. This distinction is very important. Many people struggle with mental health symptoms and are not diagnosed with a disorder. These people can still benefit from this book as a tool to reach their full potential. By design, this book will help those looking to improve their wellness and well-being, while also providing self-help tools and lifestyle interventions for those struggling with diagnosed mental illness.

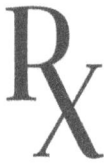

R̲X̲ 2.1 Lifestyle Psychiatry Self-Assessment

Prescription

Answer the following questions based on the last month.

Pillar 1: **Nutrition**
- a. How many servings of the following did you eat in a given day?
  - i. Meat
  - ii. Packaged foods, including processed vegetables and fruits
  - iii. Fresh fruits and vegetables
  - iv. Other
- b. Are you satisfied with your overall nutrition?

Pillar 2: **Sleep**
- a. On average, how many hours did you sleep in a 24-hour period?
- b. Was your sleep restful?
- c. Have you felt tired during the day?

Pillar 3: **Physical Activity**
- a. Describe your physical activity or movement per day, in whichever way you track it. For example, steps, miles walked, minutes exercising, times you went to the gym, yoga sessions you attended, etc.
- b. Estimate how many hours of moderate and vigorous-intensity activity you did. This will be described more in Chapter 12: Physical Activity and Movement.

Pillar 4: **Stress Management**
- a. Would you describe yourself as a stressed person?
- b. Did you set time aside each day to engage in stress-reducing practices? For example: meditation, prayer, running, etc.

Pillar 5: **Connectedness**
- a. Have you felt satisfied with your close relationships?
  - i. If not, what would you like to improve?
- b. Do you have a connection with a higher power, higher purpose or meaning in life, pets, or other connections that give your life meaning?

Pillar 6: **Substance Use Harm Reduction**
- a. Do you consider yourself addicted to substances?
  - i. If yes, which ones and how often do you use them?
- b. Do you feel the substances are affecting your functioning or quality of life?
  - i. If yes, would you like to decrease or stop using?

Rx 2.1 is a self-assessment incorporating the six pillars of lifestyle psychiatry. This Rx will serve as a starting point as you begin working through this book.

The Mental and Physical Health Connection

Fact: about 80% of chronic diseases can be prevented, treated, and often reversed with lifestyle interventions.[10]

No wonder some physicians ask about our diet, exercise, smoking, and stress, even though these questions may seem unrelated to why we're at the doctor's office.

When I was in medical school in the 1980s, we were taught that once someone had a stroke, the damage to the brain was permanent and irreversible. But now we know that's not always true! We are capable of healing and regenerating parts of our brain. This is one of the areas where the fields of lifestyle medicine and lifestyle psychiatry are gaining ground. The data is compelling—about 80% of non-infectious chronic diseases, such as type 2 diabetes, cardiovascular disease, and cancer, can be managed with lifestyle changes.[10]

While this is true for medical issues, the same principles also apply to brain and mental health disorders, such as dementia, depression, and anxiety. For example, amyloid plaques are believed to play a significant role in the pathology of Alzheimer's. Recent research has shown that these plaques may decrease with lifestyle changes and interventions like physical activity and plant-based foods.[11]

The current chronic disease crisis is intrinsically and intimately interconnected with the ongoing mental health crisis. One-third of individuals with a physical health condition are also affected by a mental health condition.[12] The number of people with chronic diseases and mental illnesses has been continually increasing worldwide.[12] The fields of lifestyle medicine and lifestyle psychiatry embrace the connection between mental health, brain health, and physical health, while also evaluating how lifestyle factors influence multiple aspects of health and overall well-being.

R⁄X 2.2 Goals for Self-Improvement
Prescription

1. What is the pillar you would like to change first?
    a. What aspect of the pillar would you like to change? For example, getting more restorative sleep, exercising more, etc.
    b. On a scale from 1-10 (1 being the least, 10 being the most), how confident are you that you can achieve this change?
        i. If your confidence is below an 8, refine your answer until you feel more confident that you can achieve a change.
    c. Are there environmental factors that are helping you or holding you back?
        i. For example, time constraints, a history of trauma, being unhoused, socioeconomic factors, or familial or social support.

For example, regular physical activity can reduce someone's risk for heart disease and dementia, while also significantly reducing their depression and anxiety levels.[13] New insights into the neural-mechanisms of health and disease have helped inform and adapt lifestyle interventions. As you consider the pillars of lifestyle psychiatry from Rx 2.1, identify the pillars you would like to change first for your own health. Complete Rx 2.2 to set your goals for self-improvement. Make sure you identify how confident you feel about making a change as well as the barriers you may face.

FIGURE 2.2 THE COMPONENTS OF LIFESTYLE PSYCHIATRY [8,9]

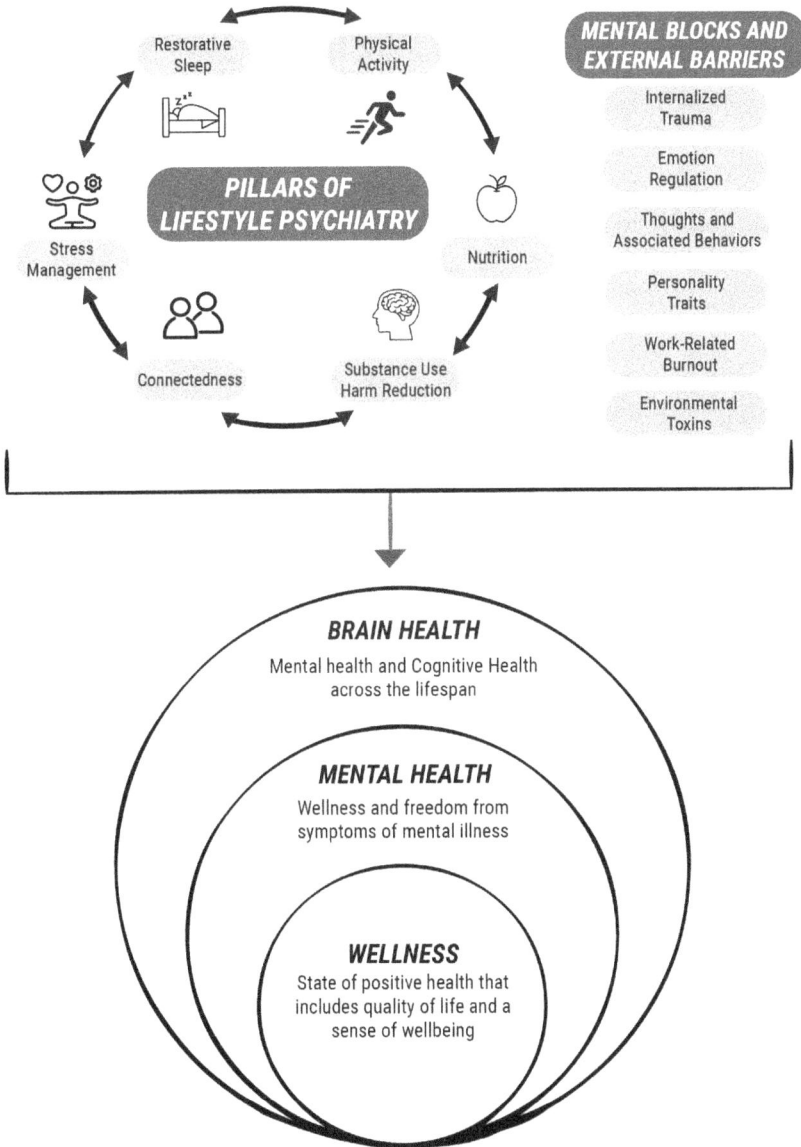

Restorative Sleep

Physical Activity

MENTAL BLOCKS AND EXTERNAL BARRIERS

Internalized Trauma

Emotion Regulation

PILLARS OF LIFESTYLE PSYCHIATRY

Thoughts and Associated Behaviors

Stress Management

Nutrition

Personality Traits

Work-Related Burnout

Connectedness

Substance Use Harm Reduction

Environmental Toxins

BRAIN HEALTH
Mental health and Cognitive Health across the lifespan

MENTAL HEALTH
Wellness and freedom from symptoms of mental illness

WELLNESS
State of positive health that includes quality of life and a sense of wellbeing

Figure 2.2[8,9] summarizes the concepts of lifestyle psychiatry, our internal blocks, external barriers and their relationship to our wellness, mental and brain health.

The Science of Brain Health

Recent advancements in brain science have better equipped us to identify and treat the root cause(s) of illness, sometimes even without prescribing medication. In recent years, with fMRI and other advanced scanning technologies of the brain available, psychiatry has become increasingly focused on brain health. The reality is the brain is the most complex and important organ in our body, and it changes constantly across our entire lifespan, starting in the fetal stages in utero.[14-16] Even in childhood, the importance of cognitive brain health is evident in attention-deficit disorders, which we can now map to regions of the brain.[17]

We're all familiar with this widely held concept: The brain is the seat of thought, and the heart is the seat of feelings. While many of us may laugh at this myth since we know that emotions do not emanate from the organ that pumps blood throughout our bodies, it seems that maybe this old concept has some merit. Feelings, though not originating in our hearts, *do* impact cardiac health. When we experience profoundly sad feelings or are grieving because of the death of a loved one, cardiac function is often affected, increasing our suffering and risk of death. In effect, our heart "feels" the sadness and the grief. I explore this phenomenon in more detail in Chapter 13: Stress Management.

Stress is a feeling state originating in the brain. Like grief, stress has also been shown to contribute to other disorders such as diabetes and cancer.[8,9] When we feel stress, we are experiencing the effects of inflammation in the brain. And inflammation can increase or decrease depending on countless factors.

Many times, people default to behaviors they think help alleviate the sensations, when actually such habits make the stress worse. Perhaps you've noticed that you gravitate toward specific changes in your diet or physical activity level when you're stressed out? It's easy, we all know, to "veg out" at the end of a difficult day in front of the TV, order unhealthy fast food, or fall back on other "easy" ways to relax. These often don't lead to restorative rest and recovery. What's needed, instead, is something like going for a jog, offloading in a journal, or taking a soothing bath.

I have been guilty of taking the easy route, too. Previously, when I had a high-pressure deadline looming, like a journal paper submission date, I would stop working out because of the time crunch. I justified skipping exercise to "buy myself" an hour or two to continue working. But not going to the gym was ultimately counterproductive. Invariably, after skipping exercise, I noticed my mood and sleep quality worsened, which compromised my ability to concentrate and be efficient. And the cycle continued! Through multiple false starts, I now have learned to do the opposite—to be very intentional about maintaining the regularity of my exercise routine during these high-pressure times. This has helped me build resilience against the impact of the stress on my body and brain.

But how can stress *possibly* have such disruptive effects on our internal systems? Well, in short, our immune system consists of a delicate balance of anti-inflammatory molecules, which decrease inflammation, as well as pro-inflammatory molecules, which increase inflammation. The brain and other cells in the body interact with and respond to the balance or imbalance of these molecules. Our lifestyle choices influence this balance and cause numerous downstream effects on our health. For example, exercise increases levels of anti-inflammatory molecules, while eating highly processed fast food increases levels of pro-inflammatory molecules.[18] Let's take a further look at how inflammation occurs in our body.

The Brain and the Gut

One of our body's systems most deeply intertwined with brain function is the part of the gastrointestinal tract that we call the gut.

The brain and the *gut microbiota*—often referred to as the gut microbiome—originate from the same set of cells in the human embryo: the neural crest. The gut microbiota refers to the diverse bacteria and other organisms located within our gut. Recognizing their common origin helps us understand the relationship between both organs. The gut and brain are connected within our bodies and communicate in multiple ways that can change throughout our lives.[19,20]

When food exits the stomach and enters our intestines, the nutrients are absorbed through the intestinal walls. We used to think that was the end of the story. But now, researchers have uncovered another key player involved in digestion—the gut microbiota.[19] In fact, the gut microbiota interacts with the brain through three main pathways: neuronal, immunological, and endocrine.

After being absorbed, food is processed and further broken down into molecules by interactions with the vagus nerve in our intestines.[21] The vagus nerve then carries information to the brain through the *neuronal* pathway. In the *immunological* pathway, other molecules, such as short-chain fatty acids, are created from food molecules that are carried by the bloodstream and can affect the inflammatory state in the body. The third set of interactions, called the *endocrine* pathway, is related to serotonin, which has further downstream effects on numerous hormones in our bodies, such as thyroid hormone and the stress hormone, cortisol. All three of these pathways—the nerves, the bloodstream, and the hormonal (or endocrine) system—circulate back to the brain.[22] Therefore, all the systems within our bodies are impacted by the foods we consume. When we choose to eat foods with ultra-processed ingredients, like a bag of potato chips, we increase inflammation in our brain and other organs in our body.

Inflammation and Our Brain

Diet isn't the only element to consider when thinking about gut health. A host of factors in our lives can negatively impact our gut health, such as too much stress, too little exercise, too little sleep, pollution in our environment, or certain medications. Given the interconnectedness of the brain and the gut described above, poor gut health in many ways can interfere with brain function.

The most common way our gut affects our brain function is through inflammation, a process that helps prepare our body for injury.[23] Inflammatory cells race to the source of the "foreign" or damaged area ready to get to work and rid the body of the offending agent. This is our natural immune response. However, if too many damaging factors—such as a poor diet, lack of physical activity, or unabated stress—accumulate, we can overwhelm our immune system with its own response mechanism.[24] A compromised immune system is no longer able to protect our body.[25] We eventually become at risk for neurodegenerative disorders like dementia, heart disease, intestinal disorders, psychiatric and mood disorders, metabolic disorders such as diabetes, and pregnancy-related complications.[26]

When a new stress appears in our life, our body's immediate response is to activate our acute nervous system response, often called the "fight-or-flight" reaction. This leads to increased blood pressure and heart rate. If the stress, or any of the contributing factors, persists long term, we may develop chronic low-grade inflammation.[27] What began as an acute problem—the inflammation resulting from stress—becomes a longer-standing issue in our bodies.[28] The inflammatory response is now no longer a one-off problem, like a one-time experience with trying cigarettes in high school. It now becomes a chronic issue like if you went to the street corner repetitively to buy drugs. However outlandish this analogy may be, let's say the drug dealer follows you back to your home and becomes your roommate, but doesn't pay their share of the rent and destroys your property. Clearly, they are an unwelcome guest—much like the inflammatory process.

Some Brain Regions of Importance in Lifestyle Psychiatry

The connection between lifestyle and the brain is depicted in Figure 2.3. We will come back to this figure multiple times throughout the book as we explore the other identified regions of the brain. While exhaustive discussions about the brain regions are beyond the scope of this book, let's discuss Figure 2.3 in detail.

The *hippocampus* is important for memory, anxiety, and stress, and may have implications in trauma and posttraumatic stress disorder. The *amygdala* is a small, complex region of the brain whose role continues to evolve over time. There are dozens of parts of the amygdala identified, all with unique functions. Parts of the amygdala play a role in the rewards system, happiness, fear, aggression, anxiety, sadness, memory, emotional learning, connectedness, alcoholism, posttraumatic stress disorder, and mood disorders. The amygdala is essential in the sympathetic nervous systems' response and has an important role in keeping the body safe. The *hypothalamus* is important in regulating our hormones in our body and especially important in controlling our food intake and our fear systems. The area of the brain known as the *septum* is located in the frontal lobe and implicated in our social behavior and memory, especially reward, motivation, and fear.

The *prefrontal cortex* is especially important in our organizational skills and planning that is associated with executive functioning, attention, and memory. The prefrontal cortex has been shown to be connected to our ability to self-regulate feelings of guilt and if damaged by injury or alcohol, it can lead to cognitive changes. The *nucleus accumbens* is in the forebrain housing many neurotransmitters such as dopamine, GABA, glutamate, and serotonin. The nucleus accumbens is part of the rewards system of the brain and is related to our ability to experience pleasure, maternal behavior, addictions, and depression.

The *ventral tegmental area (VTA)* is also part of the rewards system of the brain and is especially important in motivation, thinking, addictions, and multiple psychiatric disorders such as ADHD and schizophrenia. The *sensory inputs* are how we assimilate inputs from the external environment, including sound, vision, smell, taste, and touch. This information is then assimilated and relayed to other parts of the brain for our reactions, emotions, and can be impaired in people with sensory memories of trauma in the form of sounds, smells, etc.

Neuroplasticity and Our Brain

Our brain is dynamic and constantly evolving.

Chronic inflammation affects our brain through a neuroinflammatory process, which leads to decreased levels of substances called neurotrophic factors, one of which is brain-derived neurotrophic factor (BDNF).[29] BDNF is an example of a chemical in the brain that facilitates neuroplasticity, the brain's ability to be flexible, regenerate, and change.[30-32]

As you can imagine, if our brain's ability to change and regenerate is compromised, we'll have increased difficulty with certain basic functions like memory and learning. But more than that, BDNF and other neurotrophic growth factors operate in areas of the brain that regulate our executive function. This means that when neuroinflammation exists, we may have problems with self-control, focus, flexible thinking, working memory, and planning as well as managing emotions, feelings, and thoughts.

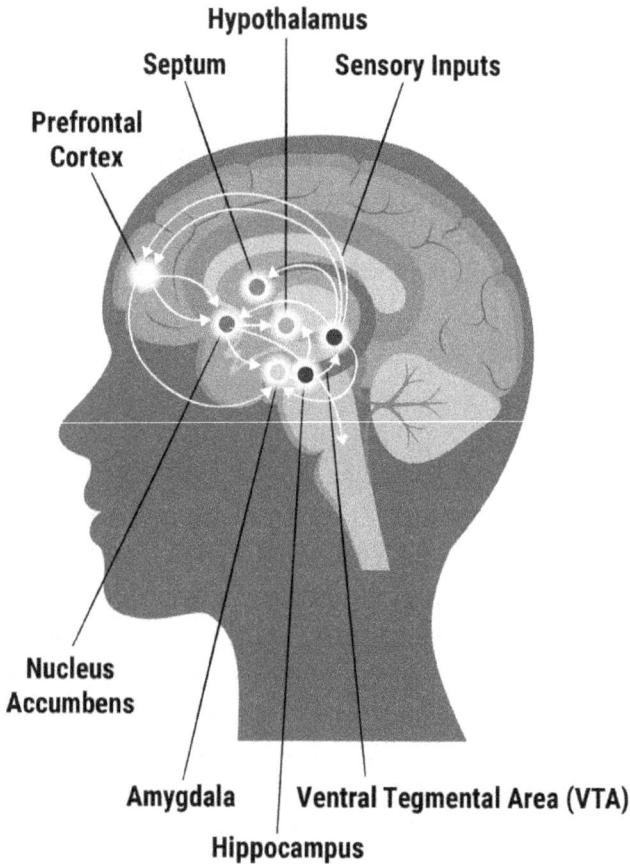

FIGURE 2.3 THE BRAIN CONNECTIONS OF LIFESTYLE PSYCHIATRY

The longer this continues, the more serious our health outcomes could be. Chronic neuroinflammation can lead to the brain aging faster and increasing risk for developing psychiatric disorders. Inflammation is part of the pathology for many medical disorders—neurodegenerative disorders like multiple sclerosis and Parkinson's disease; cardiovascular diseases like coronary artery disease and hypertension; intestinal diseases like Crohn's disease and ulcerative colitis; metabolic disorders like diabetes and obesity; and psychiatric disorders like substance use, anxiety, depression, bipolar disorder, and schizophrenia.[33-35]

Some studies have even shown an association between autism spectrum disorders and poor immune function.[36,37] Immune dysregulation in those struggling from autism spectrum disorder might be related to some of the behavior symptoms such as disordered eating, social withdrawal, and difficulty sleeping. This is an exciting area of research and helps us understand how symptoms, for example eating behaviors in autism spectrum disorder, are related to inflammatory processes.

While the science is still being worked out, neuroinflammation could be implicated in other eating behaviors as well. In fact, the changes to the brain under some psychological conditions may make patients suffer and blame themselves needlessly. If we recognize the core of the problem is something going on within the brain, we might remove some of the shame and stigma associated with people who are unable to control their eating behaviors.

In disorders that are purely medical, lab tests are used for diagnosis, and the connection between the cause and the symptoms is often clear, simple, and straightforward. An individual may say, "I took such and such medication and my labs were better," "My hemoglobin A1c got better," "My cholesterol improved," etc. However, in psychiatric diagnoses, we don't have the same precision in measuring symptom relief, as we don't have the same kinds of objective lab tests available. Still, a small lifestyle change can make a significant impact on our overall health. For example, when we don't get enough sleep, we become sluggish, and our concentration is affected. Over the long term, we're prone to becoming physically ill. We may not have lab tests to prove the correlation, but we often can trace our symptoms back and point to a lack of sleep as the culprit.

A Case of the Power of Lifestyle

Making lifestyle changes can, over time, allow us to successfully decrease or stop medications.

As an example, Mary, a 53-year-old woman and single mom of three, had many strengths, including being heavily involved within her community. Mary struggled with anxiety for two decades, and was prescribed benzodiazepines by her primary care doctor to be taken as needed. The medication helped relieve her anxiety symptoms, however, she slept only four to five hours each night. When she came to me, we first started treatment by addressing her sleep.

We discussed what she did before she went to sleep at night and ways to improve her nighttime ritual. The multiple interventions we utilized for sleep hygiene are discussed in Rx 11.2 in Chapter 11. She was encouraged to move more, beginning a regimen of walking with her friends in her neighborhood for an hour a day. This helped Mary in multiple ways, including improving her socialization, nurturing a support system, and offering a weekly dose of laughter. She started eating whole, plant-based foods two days each week, cooking in her home three days a week, and minimizing her consumption of ultra-processed foods. Within three weeks, she was using fewer of her doctor-prescribed PRN benzodiazepines, sleeping better, and came to our meetings feeling more positive about her future.

Over the next four years, we continued to improve Mary's adherence to lifestyle interventions. Because she saw positive results, she was inspired to keep up with these changes. She joined a pickleball group near her home. She became part of a bridge card game group. She never fully embraced eating an exclusively plant-based diet, but she became very plant-forward in her choice of foods. She also encouraged her friends in that direction. Eventually, she was able to completely stop the benzodiazepines. Since her anxiety had been considered mild to moderate, we were also able to stop her antidepressant medication, with no negative consequences.

Although her adherence to all the suggested lifestyle interventions was not 100% perfect, the changes she made went a long way. Ultimately, Mary enjoyed a richer life with more control over her environment and lifestyle. I have dozens of patient stories like Mary's. Perfection is not the goal.

Please note, in severe or moderately severe diseases, getting off medications is not advisable, or usually even possible. In those cases, lifestyle interventions for psychiatric disorders may allow psychiatrists to decrease doses of medication while still keeping symptoms at bay.

The Journey Ahead

Taking account of lifestyle factors contributing to our behaviors is an *oh so* underappreciated practice. We need to get to a point as a society where we understand how the foods we consume, the movements we perform every day, the stressors we're chronically affected by, and other lifestyle factors affect our medical conditions. In addition, we must accept that these components also affect our psychological health and well-being. This is especially true now that more research data points to the interrelated-ness of our lifestyle behaviors. Many in healthcare have long speculated that our bodily systems are integrated and interconnected, but now scientists are helping us see that the seat of control over all aspects of our human bodies is in the brain.

As we move to the next section on mental blocks, take some time to complete Rx 2.3 to prepare for the journey ahead. Take the Lifestyle Psychiatry Assessment (Rx 2.1), identify your goals (Rx 2.2), and make a commitment to setting goals that resonate with and will motivate you (Rx 2.3). While we will discuss many of the concepts in Rx 2.3 in detail throughout the book, putting your thoughts into writing is helpful as you set your mind on *Restack*-ing the areas troubling you. Remember, we should go back and *Restack* multiple times—*Restack* is not a singular event but an iterative process, often requiring reworking different aspects over time. Though this undertaking requires a deep dive, it is so worth it!

Congratulations. You are embarking upon a journey of self-improvement!

R͜X 2.3 Preparing for the Journey Ahead Through Behavior Change
Prescription

1. **Assess your healthy lifestyle** by reviewing your responses to Rx 2.1 Lifestyle Psychiatry Self-Assessment.
2. **Identify a goal** that you would like to achieve or work on through your responses in Rx 2.2 Goals for Self-Improvement.
3. **Make a commitment** to work through this book and make behavioral changes to the pillar you identified in Rx 2.2. Feel free to identify more than one pillar or more than one behavior you want to change.
4. **"Why?"**: Identify why you want to make changes to a specific behavior.
5. **Attitudes**: Do you have any personal stigma or social expectations towards the specific behavior you want to change? (For example, "we are a meat and potatoes family, and as such, we rarely eat vegetables or fruits" or "will I turn off my friends if I don't go out drinking with them every weekend?")
6. **Beliefs**: Do you believe that you can achieve the behavior you want to change?
7. **Habit and Routine**: How does this behavior change fit into your day-to-day? Are there other habits or routines you need to fix before being able to address this behavior change?
8. **Motivation**: What is your desire to succeed in this behavioral change, on a scale from 1 to 10?
9. **Self-efficacy**: Do you believe you have the capabilities to follow through with your goals?
10. **Intention**: On a scale from 1-10 (1 being the least, 10 being the most), how confident are you that you can achieve this?
11. **Knowledge and Skills**: Do you have the needed knowledge and skills to achieve your goals? (For example, if your goal is to change your diet, do you need to get educational material to understand healthy vs. unhealthy eating?)
12. **Journaling**: Write down your feelings and thoughts as you refine your goals.

Part B: Mental Blocks

Chapter 3: Internalized Trauma

Trauma, at its best, is a *double-edged sword* with both edges well-honed.

There is increasing awareness about trauma but some facts may be misconstrued. As such, I hope to define terms and clarify some concepts with this chapter.

Psychological trauma is usually a response to an external event, and most people don't spontaneously hurt themselves on their own or seek the traumatic external event. There are exceptions, including situations where brain changes associated with traumatic brain injuries lead to self-harm behaviors, and some neurodivergent conditions such as autism spectrum disorders. In addition, for some of us, we engage in self-sabotage or self-harm behavior without a clear connection to external trauma. Others of us may have had deaths in our families or adverse childhood experiences (ACEs) that may trigger a response. In many of these situations, though the trauma started as an *external event* or series of events, it is now taking up psychological space in our brain and is an *internalized trauma* and may be associated with mental blocks.

A Case Involving Death

I had a student, Amelia, who dreamt of becoming an oncologist, a doctor who treats cancer. During her second year of medical school, she chose a rotation on the oncology ward. Amelia overheard patients, families, and staff talk about five patient deaths during her first week on the rotation. This deeply scarred her, so much so she decided against pursuing oncology as a profession. She believed she didn't have the emotional fortitude to deal with death every day. Initially, she had been excited to become an oncologist and help save people, but the occurrence of daily deaths was not something she had envisioned.

Though her choosing not to enter this field was not a failure per se, she viewed her inability to handle her emotions around death as a personal failure, making her unqualified to be an oncologist.

Over the course of our conversations, Amelia was able to reexamine her decision and soften her self-criticism. Since Amelia was my student, my role was as a professor, not as her psychiatrist or psychotherapist. She was a woman of strong faith, so I suggested she reach out to her church to see if they offered theology-based psychotherapy. After a few visits with her pastoral counselor, she shared with me that her desire to be an oncologist for as long as she could remember. Her grandfather had died of throat cancer when she was 9 years old, and during her therapy sessions she wondered if she had been triggered by hearing conversations about death. The realization dawned on her that she hadn't really coped with her feelings surrounding her grandfather's death. She had internalized the idea that "Doctors treat people, not watch them die."

After a few more months of therapy, she felt free from the self-imposed burden of trying to cure everyone. She realized her dream to be an oncologist was born from the hope that her skills would somehow magically bring her grandfather back to life. She laughed as she told me how silly it seemed now. Amelia began finding joy in the idea of helping even one person recover in the most compassionate way possible. Ultimately, she became a truly gifted oncologist, able to relate on a deeply personal level to the pain and suffering of not only her patients, but also their families.

Amelia's emotional experience of death was raw. And the negative experiences were one edge of a double-edged sword causing her profound sadness and pain. Once she was able to grieve the death of her grandfather, she transformed that grief into her inspiration to help others. This process was foundational to building her identity as a new physician and learning how to manage potential triggering events in the future.

Psychological triggers are often seen in people who have a history of trauma. Triggers activate the hypothalamic-pituitary-adrenal axis, which results in flight, fight, or freeze responses. These responses can activate episodes of strong negative emotions, which can return people to the previous traumatic event involuntarily. Managing our involuntary responses is important not only for physicians, but for everyone. In Amelia's case, her fear of not being good enough was triggered by her exposure to death, leaving her emotionally frozen. By acknowledging and working with her trigger, Amelia was able to repurpose her traumatic experience of death into positive feelings and create a more balanced double-edged sword.

The Concept of the Double-Edged Sword

Double-edged swords, by definition, have two edges. In general conversations, when we describe something as a "double-edged sword," we often refer to a positive aspect and a negative aspect. In this book, we will be using the analogy of the double-edged sword, where the top edge represents positive emotions and the bottom edge represents negative emotions. The positive emotions are uplifting and reparative, while the negative emotions can cause distress and become overwhelming. Our goals for the two edges are similar—to identify, acknowledge, and embrace our feelings—for the positive ones, as well as the negative ones.

The secondary and more long-term aim is to build and amplify our positive experiences, in effect "crowding out" the negative ones. We can accomplish this through a variety of ways that focus on positive psychology and involve the reflective practices described later in this chapter.

Figure 3.1 shows examples of positive and negative emotions depicted on the two edges of the sword.

FIGURE 3.1 THE DOUBLE-EDGED SWORD

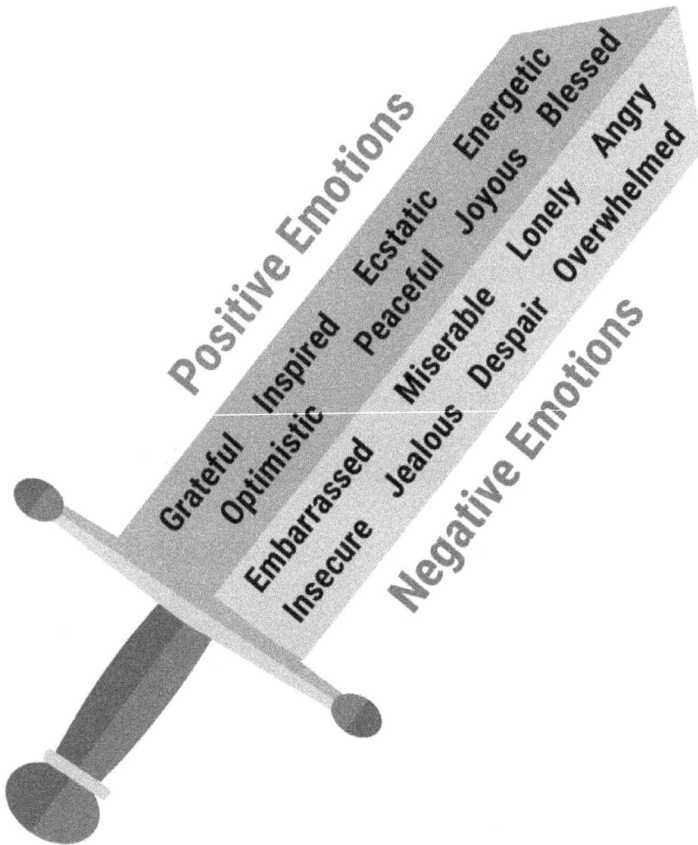

Dialectical Behavior Therapy

The concepts of positive and negative emotions and the double-edged sword draw upon a common treatment therapists use called dialectical behavior therapy (DBT). DBT helps people manage strong emotions, which is crucial to emotion regulation. The word *dialectic* means to have a conversation, which distinguishes it from another popular behavioral therapy approach called cognitive behavioral therapy (CBT). When DBT was initially developed in the 1980s by Marsha Linehan, its purpose was to help suicidal patients. Over time, DBT has been shown to be effective in much more than suicidality, including eating disorders, depression, attentional disorders, and resilience-building in schools.[38]

The Reflect and *Restack* Cycle

An experience without reflection and *Restack*-ing is a missed opportunity.

Reflection is a common word with several definitions in the English language, but it can also mean a structured process that helps us learn and grow from our experiences. This process of reflection first found its way into academic papers in the 1930s. Since then, the reflective cycle has been researched and distilled into a powerful tool for intense self-assessment. In particular, reflection is exceedingly beneficial in helping individuals after they've experienced traumatic life events. Through the reflective exercise, many people experience a feeling of regeneration, increased creativity, and, above all, emotional relief and release.[39]

While there are many structured and unstructured ways to reflect, I have refined them into the Reflect and *Restack* Cycle, depicted in Figure 3.2.[40-43] This cycle encompasses five stages: (1) describing what happened, (2) identifying your feelings, (3) considering the thoughts going through your mind, (4) synthesizing by considering other perspectives, and (5) *Restack*-ing the situation and determining how you would respond in the future.

The Reflect and *Restack* Cycle is an effective tool to use as you consider many situations in your life. An example is included in Rx 3.1, "Developing your Double-Edged Sword Through the Reflect and *Restack* Cycle."

FIGURE 3.2 REFLECT AND *RESTACK* CYCLE [40-43]

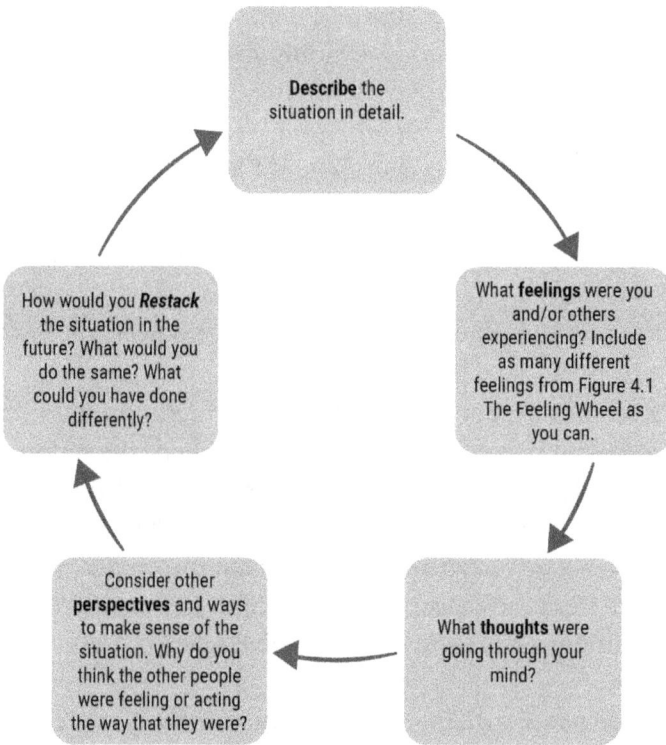

Describe the situation in detail.

What **feelings** were you and/or others experiencing? Include as many different feelings from Figure 4.1 The Feeling Wheel as you can.

What **thoughts** were going through your mind?

Consider other **perspectives** and ways to make sense of the situation. Why do you think the other people were feeling or acting the way that they were?

How would you **Restack** the situation in the future? What would you do the same? What could you have done differently?

Putting It All Together:
The Double-Edged Sword and Reflection

Rx 3.1 is an exercise to develop your double-edged sword using the Reflect and *Restack* Cycle, represented in Figure 3.2. Please complete this Rx and bookmark it, as we will continue to refer to this Rx in multiple chapters.

R̶X **3.1 Developing Your Double-Edged Sword Through the Reflect and *Restack* Cycle**

Prescription

1. Stop and consider the feelings you're experiencing when:
   a. You notice your life path has abruptly changed
   b. You want to change your life path
   c. You have a pattern you want to *Restack*
2. Use Figure 3.2 Reflect and *Restack* Cycle to critically appraise the situation.
3. Make note if you are experiencing only or mostly negative feelings.
   a. If you notice this, aim to identify positive feelings or aspects of the situation, you had not considered before. For example, if you're going through a breakup, the feelings can be overwhelmingly negative and sad. But, over time, work towards embracing the positive. The change can herald opportunities to meet new people, learn new perspectives, and connect with others who share similar interests and goals.
4. In Figure 3.1 The Double-Edged Sword add in the positive and negative feelings and aspects of the situation. The aim is to view the experience or situation through a more positive lens. Though the negative will be present, focus on buffing up a more positive lens and outlook.

A Case of Food Relationships and Triggers: My Experience

On a hot summer day in 1992, I had just finished my rounds in the hospital and was slowly meandering back to my apartment to process all that had happened that day. I was 29 years old and a newly minted resident physician, and I was still learning to manage the emotional load of the job. For me, the process of walking to my apartment involved shifting from my professional *work* self to my personal *home* self.

As I shed the doctor persona, I incrementally let my feelings in so I could deal with the stress, disappointments, pain, and reality of spending all day with people who were suffering. "Today will require a deep processing," I thought. "Maybe I need to have a long, hot soak in the bathtub."

As I approached my home, my neighbor Leslie waved me down. I had known Leslie for about a year, and we had attended several parties and dinners together. After finding out I was a psychiatrist, she disclosed to me that she had an eating disorder. The conversation got awkward. I was unsure whether she was fishing for medical advice, which I couldn't ethically or legally offer.

But that day we chatted about the weather and the new neighbors who had moved in. Nothing serious and nothing too deep. It was exactly what I needed.

Leslie usually made me tense on some level, though. She always wore makeup, even to the gym, and her hair was meticulously done. She was thin, very thin, and was getting thinner. And that day, in the 100-plus degree weather, she was dressed for the heat in attire that clearly exposed her skinny frame. I was worried about her, and I was actively managing my feelings. Clearly, she needed help. But it wasn't my role to be her physician—she had recently assured me that she was actively engaged in treatment.

Leslie was often in the parking lot when I got home from work. Coincidence? Maybe. Was she waiting here to say hello? Or, was she seeking some sort of help, hoping I would address her physical condition and discuss her eating issues? It was hard to tell.

I had to decide which person was showing up in this interaction with Leslie, my work self or my home self. As a young physician still in residency, and as someone very familiar with eating disorders, it was difficult not to feel personally involved. I entered medicine wanting to help others, but medical training and the legal aspects of medicine require physicians to hold back in many of these situations. Those boundaries need to be respected. You're only entirely free to help others when they're asking for help *and* when they are your patient. It's a hard discipline to maintain—it creates an immense cognitive dissonance—but it's necessary.

As we made small talk, another neighbor, Alan, came by and looked Leslie up and down and said under his breath, "I'd tap that." Leslie and I looked at each other, rolling our eyes, as he then blurted out, "She's hot!" Leslie turned to him with a playful smile and replied "Yes, the weather is quite warm and I *am feeling* hot." We all chuckled as his face turned red with embarrassment, and he apologized for his inappropriate outburst.

Leslie accepted the apology and I introduced them and excused myself. As I stepped into my apartment, I added another thing to my list of items to process. On the surface, I laughed it off. But in my heart of hearts, I was struggling with the concept that men found Leslie extremely attractive. She had a paper-thin physique, bones protruding everywhere, and a diagnosed eating disorder. She had mentioned to me in passing that she spends significant time in the bathroom throwing up every day. Yet she attracted men to her like a magnet.

I thought about my relationship with her. Was I jealous? I'd just had a baby a couple of years earlier. I presented a confident front, but inside I was critical of my weight, my body, and my worth, physically and in every other way. While I maintained a "normal" BMI, I had a few more curves (okay, maybe more than a *few*) than I had in high school.

During the interaction with Leslie and Alan, my thoughts centered on body weight and the dating arena. But my internal struggles were more complex. Over the next few weeks, I kept returning to that moment. I realized the issue was larger than my insecurities about how men perceived my body.

Many factors contributed to my relationship with food and my body. I had, for a long time, been using food as a source of nourishment and love. I oscillated between periods of gorging and restricting in response to my emotional state. As a psychiatrist, I found it easier to name these things than it might be for the average person and easier to identify where I needed help. Ultimately, I went through a course of psychoanalytic therapy over several years to help myself better understand the root causes of my struggles.

I received many benefits from the psychoanalysis, most importantly helping me understand myself and my patients better. I continue to use the skills I developed then with my patients now, especially when dealing with my reactions to my patients' life events, a situation therapists call *countertransference*. Countertransference is a normal human reaction, but identifying and managing it is part of the art of being a therapist. I would suggest psychoanalysis or insight-oriented psychotherapy (which is psychoanalysis "lite") for anyone who wants to understand themselves better on a deeper level. Those years of psychoanalysis helped me remove my need to be perfect and softened the hard stance I had toward myself. I began the process of practicing self-acceptance for the first time. In fact, I ended up accepting myself so completely that I started putting on weight—lots of weight.

Wait, *what*?! I healed a part of myself, then I put on weight. Yep. That's what happened.

When I quelled my desire for perfectionism, I also quelled my need to be unhealthily thin. But what didn't completely change was my internal schema—my sense of self-worth and the ability to see myself as a healthy, sexual, desirable being was not templated in my brain. When we remove the barriers to moving forward psychologically, we then must construct a *recovered* or *new* template of how to relate to the world. In my case, I had a limited internal schema for a positive relationship with food and, arguably, a positive relationship with myself.

Food had become my best friend. My sense of myself—my identity—was intertwined with the abnormal eating behaviors that had emerged after various traumas, from my childhood into adulthood. When I was 3 years old, my father had moved to the U.S. two years before the rest of my family, to complete advanced studies. It was a choice he ostensibly made for the family, but I experienced it as abandonment. Around the same time, my mother and siblings moved to a new city, and I experienced the physical and psychological loss of my nanny, who had raised me for the first few years of my life. My brother was born shortly after, demanding significant attention and energy from my mother, who herself was grappling with the absence of her husband. The combination of these losses and the isolation I experienced created attachment issues that manifested as physical symptoms in my gastrointestinal tract. For two years, I had chronic diarrhea, and multiple tests and examinations yielded no causes.

When I was 5 years old, the rest of us relocated to the U.S. to join my father, and I had to learn a completely new language and culture. I was a precocious child and had started first grade early, at the age of three. However, I couldn't grasp the rules, standards, and language of the U.S. quickly enough. I became overwhelmingly shy about eating in public.

At home, my family only ate ethnically Indian food. At school, I didn't understand what the food was, much less know the names of the items. It was an interesting disconnect between home and school. By the time I was in middle school, I had developed a habit of eating more than I should when I was lonely or feeling traumatized or struggling to cope with stressful events. I was never officially diagnosed with an eating disorder, but it became a thread throughout my life.

Many years later, as a practicing psychiatrist, I was confronted by the aggressive sexual jokes and harassment that were sometimes thrown around in medicine at that time. Progressively, in the last few decades, the tolerance for sexualized comments has diminished. But I shudder when I remember one colleague, who used to brush by me in the hallways and repeatedly and incessantly say, "I can smell your p**sy from here, it smells good. Let's hang out." I felt that I had only two options. I could choose to either be offended or to fit in and laugh everything off. I chose to laugh everything off. And, sometimes, I just walked away. I was embarrassed, and these comments affected my confidence, comfort with my sexuality, triggered fear responses, and exacerbated my struggles with my body image. I found myself eating to soothe the pain and stress. I felt I couldn't do anything about my colleagues. So, I relied on my friend—food.

One tool I used to help tease out the root of my complicated relationship with food adapts techniques from CBT, which will be discussed in detail in Chapter 16: Beyond Self-Help. While CBT is necessarily a therapy that requires a therapist trained in it for optimal results, I have borrowed principles from the CBT techniques to create the self-help version presented in Rx 3.2. This Rx focuses on one behavior, a complicated relationship with food, but it can be generalized to fit any behavior that we might want to change. For further guidance, you might find Chapter 16 useful.

R℞ 3.2 Complicated Relationship with Food
Prescription

1. Write down 4-10 aspects of your relationship with food that bother you. For example, overeating, undereating, throwing up, or emotional eating.

2. Identify how often each item of step #1 happens. For example, every minute, every hour, every day, once a week, etc.

3. On a scale from 1-10, put a number next to how much you want to change each identified aspect.

4. Do you have any of the following unproductive thoughts?
   a. Avoidance or denial
   b. Feeling that you are "fat", "too thin," or "beyond help"
   c. Feelings of perfectionism, low self-esteem, or interpersonal problems

5. Review steps #1-4 and use Figure 3.2 Reflect and *Restack* Cycle to consider the issue.

6. Replace negative and unproductive thoughts with healthier ones. For example, "My body tenses up and my hands become clenched when I'm stressed. I need food to feel calmer," can be replaced with, "I can use calming techniques to soothe myself. I don't need to overeat."

7. Continue this process of noticing and replacing thoughts.

When Self-Help Isn't Enough: My Experience

All these childhood experiences shaped my relationship with food. Though I was able to correct many of my eating behaviors with the help of psychoanalysis, I still had no healthy template to replace them.

I engaged in multiple types of therapy including CBT, self-help groups, Weight Watchers, and Overeaters Anonymous. But something was still missing. We can therapize all the trauma, remove all the barriers, heal all the hurt, but what then is available as a way of living in this world from an experiential perspective? How do we create templates in our brain as adults and find a healthy relationship with food? How do we find a way to experience our feelings when they occur, or compartmentalize them and feel them later?

One day, when I was a resident, I was walking by the ICU on my way to the outpatient clinic, when a Code Blue was called, which means there was a cardiac arrest emergency. So, I ran into the ICU and started CPR on the patient who had coded. Within the next five minutes, the rest of the team came in. I asked if anyone wanted to take over, and they said to keep going. I continued administering CPR for 30 more minutes. Then the attending physician called off the code.

The patient had officially died. I left the ICU and continued to my outpatient clinic. The first patient I saw spent the session telling me about the recent birth of their child and how ecstatic she was. My next patient talked about how his new medication was affecting his suicidal thoughts. With each of these patients, I mirrored their feelings and engaged with them in their joys and suffering. That was my job, and I did it. But I didn't get the opportunity to sit down and process the death of the ICU patient—the sadness, the guilt, the family's mourning of someone who had just barely reached middle-age, the religious aspects of his life and death—until the end of the workday.

Questions such as "What could I have done differently?" and "How would the family cope with this death?" filled my brain. An inability to compartmentalize these feelings and questions would have compromised my professional ability to provide care to my psychiatric patients. By not processing my own feelings around negatively charged events, I might be left irritable and hardened. Over time, pushing the feelings down could affect my ability to empathize with others, and potentially compromise my own mental health.

I share this story not only as a lesson about the responsibilities of a medical professional, but also as a general lesson about the need to process trauma before it gets buried beneath other events and parts of ourselves.

But how can we preserve our humanness, while maintaining an ability to function in our professional lives?

In my overeating example, I learned early in my 30s to restrict my food intake before a date or when I wanted to wear a pretty form-fitting dress that looked best with a flat stomach. This seemed to be the normative thing for every woman I knew in their 30s. At some point over the course of multiple therapies, I stopped doing that. So behaviorally, it looked like everything was fine to me and to others. I had finally conquered this problem! Right?

Unfortunately, no. All I could feel and think when I put on a dress was, "Oh you're so fat," "Oh look at this bump," "Oh look at that, if only you didn't have that cellulite there," and on and on. I would hear these thoughts and push them down, not allowing them to be experienced completely. So consciously and externally, it appeared everything was working fine. But unconsciously and internally, I was struggling. I was still dealing with memories of unresolved feelings and messages which were constantly being reinforced by my environment. The men who didn't want to go out with me. My need to be perfect, which meant my body also had to be perfect.

Don't get me wrong, the push to be perfect helped during the professional process of becoming a physician. Aspiring to perfection is something that we need in our physicians—we don't want doctors who make mistakes in their day-to-day. But for me, these memories continued to influence my relationship with food. And the deeper I pushed them, the more they became buried in my unconscious. I was less able to process the experiences and the feelings that came with them—shame, embarrassment, sadness, and loneliness. I replaced the missing emotional pieces in my life—relationships, support, and joy—with "nourishment" in the form of food.

Deep down, I was afraid of losing weight. The underlying narrative was that if I lost weight and became thin, I could be retraumatized. Staying overweight, I thought, would make me sexually unattractive, which would protect me from being hurt again. I had an intense fear of being traumatized again. Being overweight also afforded me freedom and relief from the expectations of my family. If I already didn't please them, then I could do what I wanted.

This is what we call a *cognitive distortion* in psychiatry, a specific thought pattern related to my fear of trusting the world and the rigid thinking I write about in Chapter 5. This distorted thinking, and the mental blocks it caused for me, weren't conscious. I wasn't aware I was keeping myself overweight for these reasons. But when I look back now, I can see those motivations at play.

My use of food as a friend and nourishment in this way was very adaptive, which can appear healthy on some level.

The mind succeeds in finding solutions by adapting to the situations we're in. But it can damage our body and health in the process.

Internalizing other people's expectations of us is natural and inevitable. Expressing our feelings, whether it's sadness or joy, or being triggered by an event, is also natural and inevitable based upon our life experiences. The overlay of our lived experiences is who we are. The goal is not to lose ourselves, but to maintain a healthy and balanced relationship with who we are. Throughout this book, we discuss *Restack*-ing as a goal—to *Restack* our feelings, process our traumas, and integrate ourselves in ways that preserve our uniqueness. Rx 3.3 suggests special considerations for trauma through the Reflect and *Restack* Cycle using the STOP technique commonly used in dialectical behavior therapy.[44]

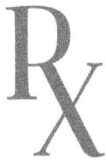

3.3 Special Considerations for Trauma Through the Reflect and *Restack* Cycle

Prescription

1. Practice the STOP Technique:[44]
   a. S : Stop what you're doing right now
   b. T : Take a few deep breaths
   c. O : Observe something in your environment, such as a body sensation, a thought, or emotion. Just be curious about what you're experiencing
   d. P : Proceed with what you were doing

2. Using Figure 3.2 Reflect and *Restack* Cycle, reflect on a traumatic event in your current life or from your past. The event could be a small or a big stressor, for example running into traffic or the death of a pet. If strong feelings emerge, go to Figure 4.2 Grounding Techniques first.

3. Once you feel grounded, go back to Figure 3.2 to write down the descriptions, feelings, thoughts, and perspectives in order to *Restack* the traumatic event.

4. Identify a trusted person to share your reflection with. This trusted person can be yourself. It can be very powerful to look at yourself in the mirror and read the reflection out loud.

The Science of Trauma

Even if we don't have a formal diagnosis, many of us can be suffering from traumatic stress.

Experiences from our childhood, adolescence, and adulthood are encoded in our brain as conscious and unconscious memories. The problem is while we may consciously get over some of our issues and problems, we may still be harboring these memories unconsciously. These unconscious traumas can shape our decisions and behaviors, or they can serve as mental blocks keeping us from reaching a fulfilling life path.

Sub-threshold traumatic events not meeting the criteria for a psychiatric diagnosis can still have long-lasting effects. In fact, I wonder if the COVID-19 pandemic was a global traumatic event affecting 100% of the world's population. So, in effect, the concepts I described in detail with my own personal life could be generalized to others in some way or another.

PTSD is the diagnosis we generally think of when we think about trauma. Recently, another term, *complex trauma*, has been added to our psychiatric nomenclature.[45] Trauma—whether it's physical, emotional, sexual, intergenerational, among others—often starts externally, but can become imprinted into our brain. Therefore, these traumas become our internal burdens.

Neuroplastic changes in our brain as a result of trauma are mostly due to the chronic effects of stress within our gut microbiota-brain axis, as described in Chapter 2.[46] During times of significant trauma, the hypothalamic-pituitary-adrenal axis is unable to downregulate the stress response, and we are left in a state of chronically high cortisol.[47] The high cortisol then causes increased release of epinephrine and norepinephrine. The fight-or-flight state that results is highly inflammatory and has been found to impair our cognitive abilities. The release of dopamine also becomes inhibited, affecting our concentration and focus. Emerging data shows people with autoimmune disorders have inflammation responses consistent with chronic trauma.[48]

The range of responses to trauma is variable. For example, people who have experienced trauma may develop avoidance or coping mechanisms to deal with the emotional pain. This may involve avoiding situations or people that serve as triggers to traumatic memories. Psychotherapy and social support systems can be valuable tools in healing from the effects of trauma, as we discuss further in Chapter 16: Beyond Self-Help.

While in this chapter we discussed trauma and ways to "buff up" our positive emotions and "muting" our negative emotions, this is a complicated dynamic requiring us to be aware of our *positive and negative* emotions and thoughts. Undoubtedly, there are some of us who need to open up to our feelings with more awareness, while others need to contain their feelings and put a lid on them. Is our ability to regulate our emotions something we can work on and get better at with practice? What techniques and tools can help us? To explore these questions, let's move to Chapter 4 and examine emotions and how to regulate them.

Chapter 4: Emotion Regulation

Art is a window to your soul—or it can be.

A Case of Expressing Feelings: My Experience

One evening, two weeks before Christmas, I stared at the empty walls of my apartment realizing I was ready to fill them with something. Paintings and pictures on a wall represent so much—they allow others to see you— to see an expression of what you believe, feel, and think.

At 29 years old, I was a single mom living in my first apartment with my then young child. I was in psychotherapy working through my traumatic marriage and divorce. Through a positive, loving, reparative relationship with my daughter, I'd gotten to a place of being able to open up and feel feelings again in a healthy way.

Over several weeks, I went from garage sale to garage sale and purchased people's discarded wall art that resonated with me. Upon putting my first painting on the wall, I burst into tears. It was a vibrant, abstract watercolor depicting joy and the possibility of happiness. As I cried, I felt an intense emotional release. I was experiencing budding feelings of love and happiness for the first time in a very long time. I had been fearful of sharing my inner life with others for so long.

In order to regulate our emotions, we need to be able to feel our feelings. For people who are blocked in their capacity to experience emotions, it's an iterative process. That is, it's a multistage process to become in tune with our feelings. Once we're able to feel them, we can then learn to regulate them. Our attempts to identify and process our feelings will be very disorganized otherwise. As obvious as this seems, we must know how to feel before we can begin to work through our feelings.

And what are feelings, anyway? We classically conceptualize feelings as an internal state. But we experience the need to externalize them—that's what the wall art meant for me. We need these windows into our psyche. The external expressions—painting, music, sculpture, dance, words—of our internal world allow others to see who we are. These expressions can also give us pleasure and serve as a way to connect with our internal states.

For years, I lived with internalized trauma. The artwork that resonated with me then was harsh and angry–pictures of blood, gore, death, dying, and suffering. This genre of art wasn't necessarily something I exclusively wanted to have on my walls. But as I changed and grew through therapy, the art I enjoyed changed with me. Now, as I write this book, I have arrived somewhere new. I find myself drawn to many pieces of art that stir uplifting positive emotions, as well as complex negative emotions.

Externalizing Our Internal States

Art can be an indirect way of externally expressing our emotions, and it's commonly employed by adults. But from a very early age, we learn to do this simply by putting our desires into motion by saying or doing what we want, or at least trying to. If we feel anger, we may yell. If we feel sadness, we may cry. As we age, we learn to manage the highs and lows of our feeling states, and the way we express them externally, through a process called *emotion regulation*. For example, a child who hears "no" may yell, scream, cry, or throw a tantrum. But over time, with *good enough* parenting, and as the child's ability to communicate becomes more developed, they will use words to express how they feel. The child will be better able to regulate the extremes of emotions.

The process of emotion regulation occurs and is made a permanent part of our patterns when we are validated, or *not* validated, by the people in our environment. The way others react to our external representation of our internal states helps mold our future reactions. If every temper tantrum a child has leads to the child being coddled, the child learns to throw temper tantrums to get what they want. Alternatively, a child who is seldom hugged or physically comforted may also struggle with soothing. In these cases, the external environment is not helping the child develop emotion regulation.

In developmental theory, the importance of an "other" in our psychological development is pivotal. We need to evolve from first identifying our feelings, to then having them acknowledged in a healthy way by someone other than ourselves–maybe by a teacher, family, guardian, or friends. In psychotherapy, this role of the therapist can be an integral therapeutic part of the process of healing.

FIGURE 4.1 THE FEELING WHEEL [49]

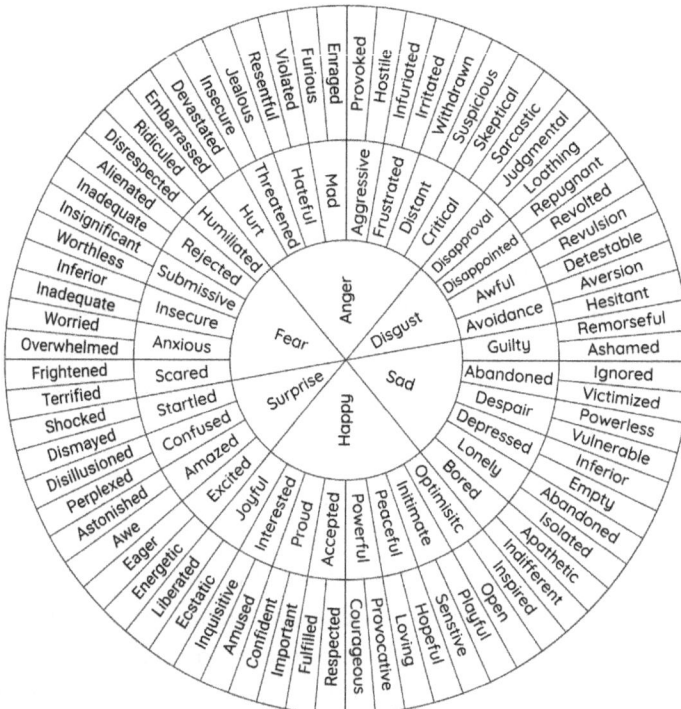

The Process of Connecting with Our Feelings

Connecting with our feelings can be broken down into multiple parts.

First, we need to notice our feelings. The Feeling Wheel in Figure 4.1 can serve as a prompt to examine our core feelings.[49] The central wheel includes the emotions of anger, disgust, sadness, fear, surprise, and happiness. While these six core feelings are easy for many of us to be in touch with, to have a complex, nuanced feeling state, often we need to be aware of when we are experiencing shades of these feelings. These shades are depicted in the outer two circles of the wheel.

Table 4.1 Common Thought Loops

Common Thought Loops	Associated Feelings
I'm so worried they will get sick.	Anxiety
I'm so stupid.	Self-criticism
I'm scared.	Trauma
Why can't they fix this?	Anger
I'll never get this done on time.	Stress
It's my fault.	Self-criticism
I'm no good.	Self-criticism
That person is too close.	Fear
I can't handle this.	Overwhelm
She's wearing THAT?	Judgment

Next, we need to identify any bodily sensations associated with these feelings. These body sensations could be pain, a burning sensation, shivering, a dull ache, numbness, tingling, etc. After allowing these sensations to be present, we should identify any thoughts associated with them. Table 4.1 lists some common thought loops which can be labeled as anxiety, self-criticism, fear, judgment, stress, or overwhelming feelings. As mentioned earlier in Rx 3.3, if we become overwhelmed with feelings or thoughts as we're connecting with our emotions or in our day-to-day, the STOP technique may be helpful. The STOP technique involves S (stopping what you're doing and thinking right now), T (taking a few breaths), O (observing and being curious about your body sensations or your environment), and P (proceeding with what you're doing).[50]

R✗ 4.1 Connecting with Your Feelings
Prescription

1. Notice your Feelings. See Figure 4.1 The Feeling Wheel.

2. Ask yourself: Are there any sensations associated with these feelings? For example, tingling, warmth, tension, etc.

3. Practice being present with emotions.
    a. Where in the body do you feel the sensations from step #2 above? For example, tingling in your fingers, warmth in your cheeks, tension in your neck, etc.
    b. Take a few moments to sit with the sensations, with your eyes closed if you are able.
    c. As you feel the sensations, be curious, kind, and non-judgmental with yourself.
    d. Thank yourself.

4. Ask yourself: Are there thoughts associated with the feelings? See Table 4.1 for examples of common thought loops.

5. If needed, practice the STOP Technique:[44]
    S: Stop what you're doing and thinking right now.
    T: Take a few deep breaths.
    O: Observe something in your environment, such as a body sensation or a thought, or emotion. Just be curious about what you're experiencing.
    P: Proceed with what you were doing.

This process of connecting with our feelings is highlighted in Rx 4.1. Connecting with our feelings may seem tedious and uncomfortable, especially to those of us who struggle in the feeling domain. But after some practice, feelings not only become easier to identify and experience, but can also bring us much joy and give us a richer, deeper, and more fulfilling life.

Coming Back into Regulation

Many of us may find we're going through life wielding the negative edge of our double-edged sword. That is, we are experiencing negative thoughts and feelings while primarily viewing things through a negative lens. Such negativity can be viewed in terms of *hyperarousal* or *hypoarousal* states. Hyperarousal states include our *fight-or-flight* response of agitation, irritability, restlessness, anger, worry, and trouble sleeping. Hypoarousal states are *freeze* responses of feeling disconnected, hopeless, exhausted, depressed, overwhelmed, and numb or wanting to be invisible.[51]

The techniques that are helpful in both the hyperarousal and hypoarousal states include engaging in physical activity, practicing the STOP technique, using the Reflect and *Restack* practices to shift our negative thoughts to positive ones, and reaching out to our loved ones. In hyperarousal states, increasing the length of our exhales while breathing helps us downregulate back to a stable arousal state. In contrast, in hypoarousal states, practicing longer inhales helps free up our *freeze* response.[50]

The goal is to get us to a more comfortable *vagal-mediated* calmness where we feel safe and connected. Vagal-mediated calmness is using our internal resources to help cope with the hyper- or hypo-arousal states. The ventral vagal state is feeling safe, grounded, present, connected, and able to access our feelings and thoughts. This is coming back into emotion regulation.[51a-c]

For clarity, the process of coming back into regulation is described as follows:

1. When you are in *fight-or-flight* mode:
   a. Someone in a hyperarousal state might experience increased sensation and emotional reactivity. For example, that person might say, "I can't calm down, my heart is beating out of my chest."
   b. Use mindfulness techniques to downregulate to a calm state. For example, calming physical activity (like yoga), connecting with relaxing people, and practicing the STOP technique.
2. When you are in *freeze* mode:
   a. Someone in a hypoarousal state might experience a relative absence of sensation and a numbing of emotions. These people might say, "I feel overwhelmed with so many responsibilities, but I have no motivation to start taking care of them."
   b. Use mindfulness techniques to upregulate to a calm state. For example, energetic physical activity (like dancing) or connecting with positive and energizing people.

Emotion Regulation in Early Childhood Development

"Don't touch that!" says the parent when a child puts their finger near an electrical socket.

Developing emotion regulation in early childhood requires numerous steps. When a 2-year-old child puts their finger near an electrical socket, often the caretaker reacts with fear and intensity. Then the child responds emotionally in a variety of ways to the caretaker's reaction. The interaction creates a psychological template in the child's mind of what is and isn't acceptable.

Early on, even when the caretaker says no, most children will repeat the undesirable behavior dozens of times because they don't have the capacity yet to fully understand "no." Once the child develops that capacity, they will stop putting their finger near the socket because of the firmness of the caretaker's voice and because the child wants to please them. Of course, children often test the boundaries of this "no" and may keep trying even if they know it displeases the caretaker. This process takes years with numerous repetitions of hearing the words and seeing the gestures of the caretaker's disapproval. Cognitive, behavioral, and emotional learning all need to happen within the child.[52]

But what is happening on the emotional front during this time? The child may have curiosity and wants to explore. They may get angry and have a temper tantrum. They may ultimately stop trying to attempt the behavior, not because they understand or agree but instead to please their caretaker. These attempts establish emotional norms and help the child understand behavioral control.

Around 3 years old, the child solidifies the ability to reason and begins understanding cause and effect. The child begins making more conscious choices, allowing them to look back at the situation, think through the process, and ultimately discuss the situation with their caretakers.[53] The caretakers can suggest safer substitutions, such as "Instead of putting your finger in the socket, why don't you play with this toy?" or, "Instead of banging on the window, take this wooden spoon and bang on the table like a drum." Through this process, the child is cognitively learning. And over time, this process will teach them self-control. Initially, the emotion regulation process is behavioral, that is, to please caretakers. As the child becomes older and their thinking develops, the process engenders a cognitive change.

At the same time that the toddler is behaviorally and cognitively developing, there are also other complex emotion processes happening.

For example, children start feeling shame, embarrassment, guilt, and pride as toddlers.[54] In fact, many toddlers can swing from one extreme feeling state to another feeling state in an instant. A caretaker's interactions with the child help them internalize acceptable emotional highs and lows. This thereby teaches the child how to regulate their feelings, including how to use words instead of actions.

The child may start understanding that when they experience a stressful event, they should talk about it or substitute healthy coping strategies for unhealthy actions or *repression*. Repression is unconsciously inhibiting or pushing down a feeling. It's also important for a caretaker to be empathetic and compassionate through phrases such as "I understand you're feeling this way." By using empathy and the consistent demonstration of rules and boundaries, a caretaker shows the child how to cope with these restrictions and how to regulate their emotions. Coping mechanisms with examples are listed in Table 4.2 and discussed in more detail later in this chapter and in Chapter 13: Stress Management.

These are all things many parents do instinctively, but it's a very nuanced interaction for the child. And at some point, even after they have learned healthy coping mechanisms, they may lose control and have a tantrum, reverting to earlier behaviors. The way caretakers emotionally respond to these behavioral tantrums helps the child understand how they ought to respond to big feelings. Children will learn from their adults. So, if we stay calm and collected, don't lose our tempers, and don't yell, then over time, most children learn they can also do things calmly.

Beyond the caretaker's emotional reaction, other helpful strategies for dealing with big emotions in a child's early development are redirecting their attention to something else (a different toy or activity), showing them affection and comfort (a hug, a kind tone, telling them you love them and know it's difficult), showing them positive reinforcement when they self-regulate so they know they've learned something valuable, and giving them choices. A child should feel in control of themselves and their environment. Instead of saying, "This is what you will eat," we can say, "Would you rather have carrots or broccoli?" "Would you rather go to sleep on this side of the bed or that side of the bed?" "Would you rather do *this* before sleep or *that* before sleep?" "Would you rather keep playing with a puzzle or put it away and read a book now?" The behavior we want to see in the child often becomes a given. In these examples, eating vegetables is a given, sleeping is a given, and winding down for bed is a given. If repeated and done consistently, the choice we give is what the child does (but, of course, some children will always resist vegetables).

By demonstrating healthy strategies for self-regulation and being consistent about boundaries and rules over the long term, we help children internalize these rules and strategies until they become templates inside their brains. The goal is that the child learns how to soothe and calm themselves. A child's ability to regulate their own emotions leads to them learning healthy behaviors. Ultimately, we want the child to be able to tie emotion regulation to healthy behaviors.

While this section has been about children's emotional development and regulation, we can extrapolate these examples to adults. Many of us still struggle with similar issues in multiple areas of our lives. Working through the Rx's in this chapter, utilizing self-talk and working with an accountability partner or a therapist can help us develop better control of our emotions.

Self-Regulation Through Coping

Self-regulation is not always automatic. We sometimes need help from learned behaviors, such as coping techniques and grounding practices.

Coping mechanisms are the thoughts and behaviors we use to deal with negative emotions and stressful situations in our lives. The way we cope can be categorized as either leaning toward being more positive or more negative. Coping strategies are usually not black and white but are conceptually on a spectrum. The most positive coping strategies include positive cognitive restructuring, problem-solving, and seeking support. The most negative coping strategies are escape and avoidance, whereas distracting ourselves can be placed in the middle. Table 4.2 lists coping mechanisms and their definitions, with examples.[55]

Table 4.2 Coping Mechanisms[55]			
Categories of Coping	**Positive or Negative?**	**Definition**	**Examples**
Positive cognitive restructuring	Most positive coping strategy	During a stressful situation, actively taking a more optimistic lens.	Seeing the glass half full, flooding out the negative thoughts with the positive, using positive psychology techniques, being optimistic.
Problem-solving	Most positive coping strategy	Using strategies to resolve situations to have a better outcome.	Planning and analyzing, remaining persistent and determined through the process.
Seeking support	Positive coping strategy	Reaching out for help from social network and other connections in the community.	Any form of connectedness (Chapter 14), including from family, partners, friends, work colleagues, God, or a higher power.
Distraction	Can be positive or negative	During a stressful situation, shifting one's attention to focus on another activity.	Positive distraction includes taking a break, watching TV, exercising, or participating in hobbies. Negative distraction includes unhealthy substance use.
Escape/avoidance	More negative coping strategy	Avoiding painful or unpleasant situations that are related to the stressor.	Forgetting the painful situation as in trauma, socially isolating, experiencing excessive sensitivity to stressful events.

FIGURE 4.2 GROUNDING TECHNIQUES

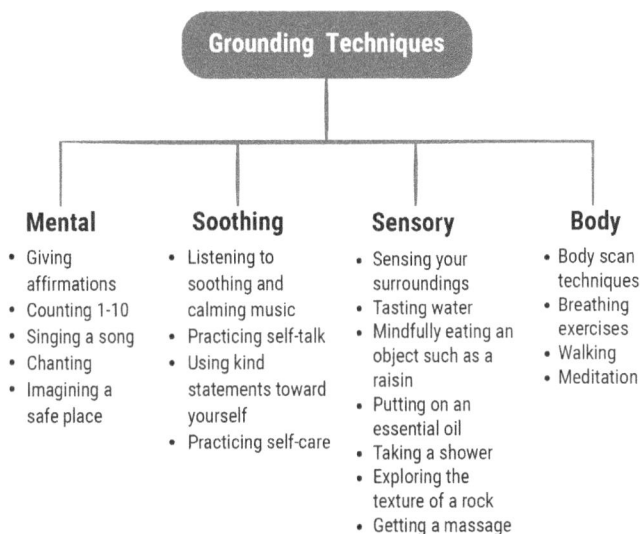

Grounding Techniques

Mental
- Giving affirmations
- Counting 1-10
- Singing a song
- Chanting
- Imagining a safe place

Soothing
- Listening to soothing and calming music
- Practicing self-talk
- Using kind statements toward yourself
- Practicing self-care

Sensory
- Sensing your surroundings
- Tasting water
- Mindfully eating an object such as a raisin
- Putting on an essential oil
- Taking a shower
- Exploring the texture of a rock
- Getting a massage

Body
- Body scan techniques
- Breathing exercises
- Walking
- Meditation

Self-Regulation Through Grounding

We hear people described as "well-grounded," but do you know what it means as a way of regulating our emotions?

Grounding involves techniques that help us get in touch with our senses. These strategies help us regulate our emotions, respond to stress, and calm ourselves. Grounding techniques can be broken down into four categories: mental, soothing, body, and sensory.

Mental grounding includes practices such as using affirmations, singing a song, and counting from 1 to 10 before taking an action. Soothing activities entail using positive self-talk, speaking kind statements to others, and engaging in self-care. Body grounding is as practical as it sounds and includes body scanning techniques—such as bringing attention to parts of our body while our eyes are closed—as well as meditation and breathing exercises. Lastly, sensory grounding includes applying essential oils, taking a shower, getting a massage, and focusing on the taste of foods. Figure 4.2 lists several grounding techniques. Note that certain tasks or practices may fall into multiple categories.

The Building Blocks of Self-Regulation Exercise

Using the coping strategies and the grounding techniques together can be a powerful way to start building our self-regulation skills. In Rx 4.2, first identify your feelings using The Feeling Wheel in Figure 4.1. Then, choose positive coping mechanisms from Table 4.2. Finally, use the grounding techniques in Figure 4.2 to help you regulate your mind and soothe yourself.

R̶X 4.2 The Building Blocks of Self-Regulation
Prescription

1. **Identify your feelings.** Refer to Figure 4.1 The Feeling Wheel.
    a. For example, suppose you're feeling worthless because your supervisor gave you a negative review on your job performance or you scored poorly on an exam.
2. **Use positive coping mechanisms.** Refer to Table 4.2 Coping Mechanisms.
    a. From the table of coping mechanisms, consider ways you could positively restructure the situation. Using the example from step #1, how can you cope with your feelings and move forward? Some options include engaging in a conversation with your supervisor for constructive feedback, or considering if this is a job you're passionate about or if you want to explore other options. Similarly, if you scored poorly on an exam, you may want to reach out to peers or the instructor for tips on how to study for the next exam.
3. **Use grounding techniques.** Refer to Figure 4.2 Grounding Techniques.
    a. In this example, suppose you identify feeling a lot of performance or test anxiety. Using Figure 4.2, identify grounding techniques that may help you, like breathing exercises and affirming self-talk.

Emotion Dysregulation in Adults

Which is harder: feeling too little or feeling too much?

I've spent many years trying not to feel sadness for every downtrodden person or animal I encounter. In the past, my empathy led me to repeated thought loops, with trouble disengaging my own thoughts from the suffering of others. Even now, I often feel my heightened level of emotional connection to the world is a curse. But would turning a blind eye to someone's suffering and not feeling their pain be a better way to go through life? And if this heightened empathy and compassion for others is part of the lens I view the world through, how might it interfere with my personal and professional life?

At some point, I got so mired in feeling the pain of others and, in fact, feeling my own pain that I was unable to function. I was drowning in a pool of pain. Earlier in this book, I mentioned not being able to feel much at all, and the subsequent joy from getting back in touch with my emotions. My body may have blocked my feelings as a protective mechanism against experiencing pain at all.

In ideal situations, we create the upper and lower bounds of emotional experiences through our early development. But if our environment doesn't communicate to us (in a healthy way) what is and isn't healthy behavior, we develop problems with regulating our emotions. This is simply called *emotion dysregulation.*

To illustrate this term, if our caretakers acquiesced to our refusal to brush our teeth every night, we would not have developed the structure in our brain and the habit of daily dental hygiene. Many of us who learned these behaviors early on don't even think twice about brushing our teeth. But many also may have missed some of these lessons (such as washing our face, flossing, exercising every day, or eating healthy foods) for a myriad of reasons, ranging from the cultural to the economic.

In the same vein, if our templates for healthy coping strategies aren't firmly established, then during times of stress or intense emotional upheaval, we may lack the tools to internally regulate our emotions and thus may resort to unhealthy coping strategies. Ultimately, creating healthy habits and developing healthy coping strategies points back to emotion regulation. If this is something you struggle with, then the Rx's in this chapter may be worth practicing regularly and with intention.

As a note, some individuals who are neurodivergent may inherently struggle with regulating their emotions, not due to lived experiences in early childhood.[56] Examples of neurodivergence include autism spectrum disorders, ADHD, dyslexia, and Down's syndrome. More recently, some authors have included all diagnosed mental health disorders in the neurodivergent category. So, what I am highlighting is that though the patterns established with caretakers in early development are a piece of the puzzle, some of the emotion dysregulation we experience may be due to our other factors not related to early interactional patterns. The techniques described in this book can still be used for these obstacles and are often among the tools clinicians use during therapy for many disorders no matter the cause.

A Case of Working Through Mental Blocks: My Experience

As I mentioned in previous chapters, I often used overeating as a coping strategy for stress. Food became a very available, easy *friend*. This behavior was maladaptive, in every sense of the word.

Whenever I felt big feelings, I turned to food. And interestingly, over time, I wasn't even experiencing big feelings anymore. I didn't feel the stress or negative emotions in my day-to-day, but they were still there. I just wasn't conscious of them. They were present on an *unconscious* level. When I ate to soothe myself, I wasn't thinking about coping—it just became a habitual behavior to eat excessively.

For me, going to Weight Watchers or other weight-management programs worked for the time I attended. I addressed the behavioral aspects of my overeating, and my behaviors changed. But they didn't stick because the emotional templates informing the behaviors hadn't been changed or relearned—the *Restack* wasn't complete. The architecture in my brain needed reworking too. Such reworking can take years of repetition or using a different approach so that all aspects of the issues are addressed. My response to stress, which wasn't even conscious anymore, was still to overeat. On top of that, I experienced enormous shame for not losing weight despite all my trying, which then perpetuated the self-criticism loop and triggered more emotional overeating.

Interestingly, my relationship with exercise and physical movement has also been problematic throughout my life partially because of some of the templates I internalized concerning exercise during my early childhood.

I grew up in an Indian family, and at times, we would excitedly go to watch Bollywood movies that would screen a couple of times a year in the city since DVDs and streaming services didn't exist yet. It was a fun, social event with families coming together to see recently released Indian movies. One advertisement that consistently played during intermission stood out to me the most. It was about a skin whitening cream called Vicco Turmeric, which displayed a before and after picture of a woman with dark skin becoming light skinned. I came to learn that, in India, light skin was more desirable and could affect a woman's value during an arranged marriage. Vicco Turmeric had a lot of loyal consumers who I think bought it in bulk. Arranged marriages were an important rite of passage at that time.

Watching that commercial and absorbing the cultural mores that it suggested, I was dumbstruck. The previous summer, when I was 8 years old, I had almost become pitch black after spending the whole summer at the neighborhood pool. Did people find me unattractive? Was I ruining my chances of getting married? And a more immediate concern, as a budding pre-pubescent girl, would I ever find a boyfriend? As an extremely sensitive child who wanted to be liked and considered attractive, the next summer I avoided the sun. The pool was no longer a fun place to be. My days were filled with sitting inside, playing with toys and dolls by myself. So, the normal physical activities—playing games, running around, swimming, jumping in the pool—did not only feel unavailable to me, but I also developed negative associations with them. I felt I was being a bad girl if I engaged in those activities. I lost out on the benefits of that socialization, joy, and fun.

Children at that age misrepresent and misinterpret the realities of the outside world in a very egocentric way: They assume they caused the problem. That's how I felt—I assumed that I was flawed because I tended to get very dark very fast. I lived in almost exclusively white neighborhood in Louisiana, and I believed that the beauty standards necessarily were for my skin tone to stay as light as possible. We had two races back then, White and Black. I passed as a White girl until the summer.

Over time, my flawed thought pattern and my reality ate at me. I struggled with the consequences of having distant relationships with kids my age, due to my isolation during the summers. I did adapt and develop friendships with other children who also couldn't take advantage of these outdoor opportunities, but in my heart, I wanted to be active and out playing in the sun.

Thinking about my distorted perceptions now, I know I was doing the best that I could. Was my avoidance of outside play because of social anxiety, the desire to please the Indian community at large, or from a fear of becoming "too dark" and being rejected by my friends? Probably all of them in some way. Yet, I was conflicted. To this day, I remember with longing and sadness the medals my brother won on the swim team those summers while I forced myself to stay indoors.

In my adulthood, I often felt a constant pull to avoid outdoor activities and the sun. While this is a mental block, I am sure that dermatologists would appreciate my aversion to tanning since any amount of tanning can increase your risk of cancer. I love playing tennis, but I always look for indoor tennis groups to play with. I tend to go to the pool only after 6 pm. And though I love going to the beach (with adequate sunscreen!), I have to remind myself that not becoming tan doesn't make me a lesser human. I'm able to overcome that internal criticism with grounding techniques and self-talk. But the dialogue is still present. The jingle "Vicco, Vicco Turmeric" still lives rent-free in my brain, showing itself at the first sight of the sun in the spring. I now smile and say to myself, "It's okay," and move on.

Tanning has many meanings across various cultures. In the Western world, mostly among fairer-skinned people, going to the beach and comparing the quality of their darkened skin is a symbol of summer fun and privilege. However, in many cultures, laborers who work outside in the sun, which results in darker skin, are often seen as being lesser-privileged humans. To be sure, in some cultures, a tan is not a badge of honor, but a branding of the working class.

I have been very intentional about changing this cultural pattern by teaching my daughter as she was growing up that color is beautiful and encouraging her to be outside. It brought me so much joy to watch her go to the backyard to play while she was in middle school, while using proper protection from the harmful ultraviolet radiation, of course. And now, I revel as I hear her say, "Dark is beautiful," to her son with such assuredness, in a way that carries forward and heals not only my history, but also our cultural history.

Just as it takes a long time and a lot of consistency to establish templates of behavior in early childhood development, it also takes a long time and much intention to replace those templates when they are harming us. Sometimes, these templates cannot be easily replaced—these mental blocks may feel fixed and immovable. In this case, we may need to learn how to deal with these mental blocks in the most gentle and loving way. Our job is to become aware of the triggers so we can employ healthy coping strategies as we continue to improve our relationship with our emotions.

With awareness, we can continue to *Restack* the emotions, behaviors, and coping strategies whenever they are holding us back, while showing ourselves grace.

Creating and Maintaining the Double-Edged Sword of Positive and Negative Emotions

How do we create that balance of positive and negative emotions?

In the last two chapters, we have been discussing emotions and our responses to them. As described in Chapter 3, the double-edged sword of positive and negative emotions can be a powerful way of visualizing our internal feelings. Regulating and maintaining our emotions requires multiple steps.

First and foremost, we must be able to recognize our feelings. These may be primary feelings we experience or secondary feelings in response to others. We then can create goals and actionable steps through the Reflect and *Restack* Cycle in Figure 3.2. This is crucial to understanding how these habits affect our well-being. Identifying our emotions and the patterns of thinking that get in our way are important aspects to be aware of as we try to cognitively restructure through the CBT techniques described in Chapter 3.

Throughout this process, we need to self-validate, accept our emotions, and focus on replacing unhealthy thoughts with more helpful and positive ones. Imagining scenarios and rehearsing them in our head leads to an improved ability to cope with challenges we may face. In Rx 4.3, these steps are laid down as a prescription.

R/X **4.3 Emotion Regulation Through The Double-Edged Sword: Putting It All Together**
Prescription

- **Recognize** your primary and secondary emotions.
- **Set goals** (both short- and long-term) and define actionable steps to reach the goals.
- **Assess** how your behaviors influence your well-being.
  - Identify what your current behaviors are and how you want to improve them.
- **Identify** your emotions and patterns of thinking.
- **Accept** your emotions through self-validation.
- **Bust any myths** you have about emotions.
  - For example, replace "I shouldn't let anyone else know how I feel because then they'll think I'm weak" with "Emotions are how we react and they're normal. Just because I express something doesn't mean I'm weak."
- **Avoid blocking** negative emotions.
  - Feel your emotions and learn how to cope with them without denying them, in order to get past them.
  - **Pinpoint** and address potential triggers.
- **Create a balance** of emotions by flooding yourself with positive feelings. Figure 3.1 The Double-Edged Sword can be used as a tool in buffing up the top edge of the sword.
- **Practice problem-solving and coping** through imagining problematic scenarios and preparing to deal with them in the future.

The Science of Emotions

Data shows that the multi-billion-dollar weight loss industry is rarely successful in helping dieters sustain weight loss one year later.[57] Recently, with the surge in use of GLP-1 medications for weight loss (like Ozempic) there have been many success stories. Of course, everyone has to evaluate the benefit for themselves given the potential risk of adverse effects. What happens when someone stops taking the medication? Have the diet and habits changed enough so as to not put significant weight back on? While the medical community continues to debate the side-effects, the long-term risk of weight gain, and the unknowns concerning these drugs, focusing on lifestyle changes that would help sustain the weight loss over time seems like a sound investment in personal health.

The amount of mortification and embarrassment many of us feel leaves us discouraged, hopeless, and at times suicidal if we fail to lose or regain weight. We are often left to wonder how we can be so smart, capable, and bright in our work and our lives, yet we can't control this one thing.

For example, many people often feel worse about themselves, sometimes becoming clinically depressed, when their weight *yo-yos*. In fact, well-meaning acquaintances, experts, and friends can do more harm than good with their words. For example, some dieting gurus focus on motivation/drive, commanding dieters to: "Just do it. Just stop eating so much." This ridiculous oversimplification minimizes how entangled our weight loss issues are with our psyche. This reductionist attitude of some self-motivation gurus can be experienced by many of us as insulting and indicates their misunderstanding of human nature. To be sure, we are in a crisis of people struggling globally with weight-related issues. Estimates are that 20% of children under the age of 10 in the U.S. are struggling with being overweight or obese.[58] As a culture, we're overfeeding and overeating. Though a simple "just stop eating" may be said with care and concern, it often misses the mark.

The science of what happens during emotional eating is similar to addiction theory for substance use disorders.[59] Eating behaviors and addiction are both regulated in the brain by a complex series of reward pathway interactions between dopamine, the mesolimbic network, the prefrontal cortex, and the nigrostriatal network (see Figure 2.3).[60,61] Eating ultra-processed or high sugar food produces very elevated levels of dopamine, much like those triggered by recreational drugs, for example.[61] Because of this, it's easy to develop addictive behaviors in relation to these foods. For those of us who are vulnerable to addiction, our brain interacts with them in the way it would interact with a party drug.

What this means is, as an addiction, we usually just can't decide to "stop." That answers the question of why sometimes the well-meaning phrase, "Just stop eating," doesn't work. It's like telling a person who is using fentanyl to "Just stop doing drugs." We know that very few people who are misusing substances can stop cold turkey. They often need to get treatment, and recovery is a multistep process.

Just like addiction treatment requires continued work, so does emotional overeating. The process involves changing our intentions and behaviors around food. As with an individual struggling with alcohol use disorder, an emotional overeater may need to avoid a triggering substance (chocolate, for example) and remove it from their home. Most emotional eaters know this well—once they start eating their triggering food, they can't stop. But, also like the individual with alcohol use disorder, once the compulsive behavior is under control, the urges will reduce significantly over time, as well as the amount of energy required to maintain sobriety or maintain healthy eating behaviors.

Another helpful approach has come from the Alcoholics Anonymous world and has been adapted by many therapists. Often, therapists recommend not engaging in the unhealthy behavior when we are hungry, angry, lonely, and tired—the acronym of which is HALT.[62]

The path forward for many of us who are suffering often includes fostering the courage and vulnerability to acknowledge that our behaviors and thoughts are connected to our emotions.

The Connection Between Feelings and Thoughts

Thinking about our feelings is satisfying—but *feeling* them is even better!

Being able to *feel* our feelings is important for optimal human emotional development. While behavioral and cognitive adjustments are necessary, we still need to rework our emotional relationship with the behavior we want to curb. Back to the example of eating, this involves refining what we consider pleasurable. If we associate pleasure with things that are unhealthy—ultra-processed, high-sugar foods, for example—we have to remove this association and find something healthy we can associate with pleasure.

The best way to do this is to identify *why* we want to change. Perhaps we've developed diabetes, or maybe we feel sick or constantly bloated, we have chronic constipation, or we must take medication to manage a condition or disorder. These are all good reasons to want to change our eating behaviors. Our first step is to associate these negative consequences with the unhealthy foods we may be craving. After that, we can establish connections between consuming healthy foods and positive ideas or feelings. We must remind ourselves that this new positive association is healthy and empowering, helping us to feel good. Or more than that, we can tell ourselves we want to live longer, perhaps to see our children grow up or enjoy our retirement.

Something that can be very helpful on this front is to have these positive and negative associations reinforced by someone else—a coach or an accountability partner or anyone who carries influence in our lives. An *accountability partner* is someone who provides us support and helps us maintain focus toward a desired goal. Working with another person can be a very powerful tool in our commitment, one that provides us with external validation as we work to change our behaviors. After all, that's how we developed an emotional template in relation to eating in the first place—with an external person or source validating us! We need that same external interaction to form a new template. In order to enter into these interactions and rewire our emotional templates, we have to be open-minded. Likewise, in order to associate the new behavior with our emotions, we must allow ourselves to be vulnerable, to show our internal lives to others, and to express our values.

As described earlier, I was finally able to place art on the walls of my apartment. But that action is not the end of the journey—it's the beginning. Accepting the placement of art in my home, physically putting it on the walls, got me to a point where my internal feeling states were available to be worked on. For others, the process may start with putting words to feelings. What is the whole journey? In my case, the path forward involved many small steps over many years. Emotion regulation is an iterative process, a series of gradual changes, such as developing openness to change, practicing optimism, regulating our stress, and connecting socially with others, among other things. We're going to continue to talk about that process throughout the book.

The building blocks of *Restack*-ing include practicing the grounding techniques, recognizing our feelings, coming back to emotion regulation, and employing positive coping strategies. This chapter was all about feelings and their associated behaviors. But what happens with our thoughts? For those of us who are mostly "in our heads" and lead with our thoughts, how do we address getting in touch with our feelings? What is the complex dance between our feelings, thoughts, behaviors, and our bodily sensations?

Chapter 5: Thoughts and Associated Behaviors

It was a typical Thursday morning during the first week of my emergency psychiatry rotation at University of Texas Southwestern Medical Center in Dallas, TX. As a first-year resident, I was required to present my patients to the attending psychiatrist, Paul Mohl, for supervision.

John Doe was a 50-year-old male who came to the emergency room with no wallet, no shoes, and no identifying information. John Doe was mumbling to himself and seemed out of touch with reality. It was unclear how he got this way. I didn't know what to do.

After my presentation, Dr. Mohl turned to me and asked, "How do you feel?"

I took a step back and said, "This is a complicated situation."

Dr. Mohl repeated, "How do you feel?"

I replied, "I think it's important for us to figure out who he is."

Dr. Mohl asked again, "How do you feel?"

I responded, "I think his nails are clean, and there's no dirt in them. Maybe something happened, like a car accident or a stroke, and he's not able to relay that information to us."

Dr. Mohl looked at me with a questioning gaze. "So, I asked you three times about how you felt, and you told me what you thought."

It was one of the most confusing statements I had heard from one of my supervisors since starting my residency. And this comment has stuck with me all these decades. When I began my residency, my thinking was clear, logical, and usually spot-on. But my feelings? I had no concept of my feelings being important in the profession. Dr. Mohl's lesson, though gently spoken, was a hard one for me. As an astute psychiatrist, he quickly identified one of my biggest weaknesses, and one I continued to work on for years.

I now think back on John Doe. At the time, I *felt* scared, I *felt* vulnerable, and I *felt* frightened for this man. I *felt* he could've been my relative and just came upon hard times and needed my help. I worried that he was someone's loved one and they were desperately searching for him and that it was my job to solve the mystery of who he was. I needed to learn how to manage my strong feelings to take care of him, but at the same time, not be intimidated by his physical appearance. There could've been so many causes for his cognitive state and his disheveled appearance.

I was focusing exclusively on my thoughts when discussing John Doe, and I needed help getting in touch with my *feelings* about his state. Years of medical school had helped me learn the languages of facts, analysis, and monotonous memorized concepts, but hadn't mentioned how my feelings factored into the treatment process. I had absorbed this detached approach to the point that while sitting in anatomy lab, dissecting a woman's body with unabashed eagerness, I lost touch with the human she had been when she was alive.

Before medical school, I was a person who recoiled at the sight of blood. I would get a heavy feeling in my stomach whenever I saw dead animals on highways. My empathy colored the lens I saw the world through. The further I got into my training, however, I realized these emotional responses to death had to be tucked away so I could do the work of a medical student and continue to learn. I became an expert in compartmentalization.

As you reflect on your life and your responses to situations, are you more of a thinking person or an emotional person? Do you automatically focus on the cognitive aspects of a situation? Or do you stay with the feelings?

Either extreme could be problematic. Ultimately, the goal is to have both thoughts and feelings available for us to draw on, though any single situation may require a unique combination of these two approaches.

Feelings, Thoughts, Behaviors, and Bodily Sensations

There is a delicate dance between our emotions, our thoughts, our bodily sensations, and our subsequent behaviors, but they are separate processes in our brains.[63-65]

In the previous chapter, we discussed emotions, feelings, and the subsequent thoughts associated with them. In this chapter, we are continuing the conversation forward and considering these thoughts and feelings as primary mental blocks. We are drilling down to understand them better and how they affect our behavior.

In my conversation with Dr. Mohl, I confused my feelings with my thoughts. So how do we develop clarity about the differences between feelings, thoughts, behaviors, or bodily sensations?

In Figure 5.1, if we use "cooking healthy food" as an example, how can we express these four different components in words? The thoughts might be, "I want to cook some healthy food today." The feelings could be, "I feel guilty about all the fast food I've been eating lately." The resultant behavioral action could ultimately lead to cooking the healthy food. In addition, we often need to acknowledge any bodily sensations that can arise during this process. For example, we may experience low- or high-energy states, tension, or heart palpitations. If our feelings are hard to identify, focusing on our bodily sensations can give us information about our mental blocks. These separate components are all interrelated, as is noted by the arrows in Figure 5.1.

FIGURE 5.1 RELATIONSHIP BETWEEN FEELINGS, THOUGHTS, BEHAVIOR, AND BODILY SENSATIONS

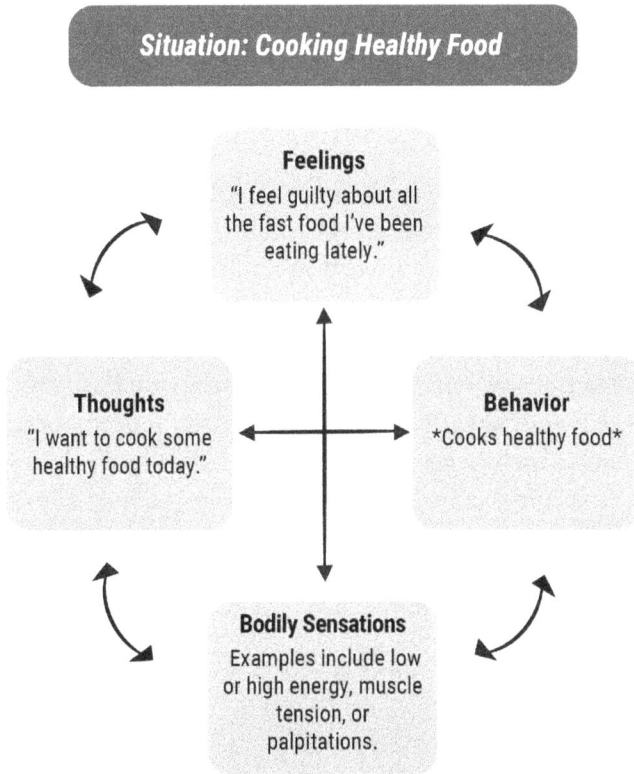

Situation: Cooking Healthy Food

Feelings
"I feel guilty about all the fast food I've been eating lately."

Thoughts
"I want to cook some healthy food today."

Behavior
Cooks healthy food

Bodily Sensations
Examples include low or high energy, muscle tension, or palpitations.

We discussed this interrelation in Chapter 3, Figure 3.2, the Reflect and *Restack* Cycle, where we stressed working through our feelings and separating them from our thoughts in any given situation. This is important since solely focusing on feelings or thoughts can lead to imbalances and mental blocks in our responses to situations. Rx 4.1 in Chapter 4 also encouraged connecting with your feelings. This was what first-year-resident-physician-me needed in order to get in touch with my emotional response to John Doe's plight.

As clinicians, not being in touch with our feelings can lead to very robotic responses to our patients, stripping us of the joy in the human connection that gives our job meaning. More importantly, patients can sense this distance in their clinician, which can lead to an unsatisfactory experience. For the non-healthcare professional who approaches life more by thinking than by feeling, a consequence of a similar process may be suppressing what gives life its meaning and makes us human.

Our Cognitive and Behavioral Responses

We can fully understand something—our emotions and our thoughts—but it's a missed opportunity if we don't take action.

Cognition refers to our internal processes of thinking. Behavior refers to our external actions. Often, cognitive and behavioral are used together, since having an understanding of our thoughts is helpful, though putting them into action usually gets us where we want to be.

Behaviorism was first noted in the 19th and 20th centuries in the U.S. as a movement away from psychoanalysis and deep internal searching for the meaning of behavior.[66,67] As described in Chapter 16: Beyond Self-Help, not every field of psychiatry, nor every clinician, looks at solutions the same way. Indeed, the field of evidence-based psychiatry branched out from behaviorism in the 1960s to treatments such as cognitive behavioral therapy and dialectical behavior therapy. Ultimately, all these treatments emerged from the earlier work of psychoanalysis, and now in the 21st century, we are incorporating insights from brain science.

While behavior and our thinking are valid and important aspects of the overall *Restack*-ing of ourselves, sometimes we have to go deeper and make those connections that transcend just our cognition. Potential trauma, social determinants of health, and our work environment may all be relevant to our *Restack*-ing. To move forward we may need to connect with our emotions and remove any mental blocks. While habits are important, they are only part of the equation.

Table 5.1 Definitions and Examples of Common Cognitive Terms and Processes		
Term	Definition	Examples
Cognitive distortions	Thoughts, beliefs, or perceptions that are not accurate. While cognitive distortions are normal, the extent to which they occur may become problematic.	"I'm *always* making mistakes and disappointing others." "It's *impossible* for me to make friends."
Thought loops	Thoughts that recur over and over again. These are commonly seen in anxiety (without a diagnosis), but are also seen in anxiety disorders and obsessive-compulsive disorder.	A new mother's internal dialogue ("remember that the baby needs milk every 2 hours") to make sure she feeds her newborn enough. While this thought loop could be normal, it could also lead to a diagnosis of anxiety disorder if the thought loop is extreme.
Cognitive dissonance	A mental state of having two different (and often conflicting) thoughts, values, and beliefs. Usually occurs after new contradictory information is presented when we already have a fixed belief.	Thinking: "I'm improving my health on a keto diet," and then reading Chapter 10: Nutrition and realizing meats and ultra-processed foods are associated with many negative health outcomes.
Cognitive restructuring	Identifying our negative beliefs, labeling the negative beliefs as cognitive distortions, mentally disagreeing with the negative beliefs, and modifying them to more positive/healthy/adaptive responses.	In the case of depression: 1. Negative belief: "No one likes me." 2. Labeling and mentally disagreeing with the negative belief: "I am a likable person," "I may not feel like I have friends right now since I've been staying home all day." 3. Modifying the belief to a more healthy response: "I am worthy of having friends," "I can find more people to be friends with," "I know people who care about me."

Working with Our Thoughts

Having a lot of thoughts doesn't necessarily translate to *useful* thoughts or actions.

In Table 4.1, we discussed common thought loops that may be blocking our connection with our feelings. We are now going to take this a step further and examine the process of changing our negative thoughts through the cognitive techniques clinicians use with patients.

Cognitive behavioral therapy (CBT) was first developed by Aaron Beck in the 1960s. CBT is a manualized, structured approach to treatment with a licensed clinician.[68] Manualized means that, by design, the treatment must necessarily be done with a clinician who is trained in the formal protocol of CBT. What I am describing in this book is not CBT but techniques that are rooted in CBT.

To get us all on the same page, let's review some commonly used cognitive terms and processes with examples in Table 5.1.

Using the Thought Ladder and Action Roof Exercise

According to a 2020 research study using the latest fMRI scanning techniques, it's estimated that we have about 6,500 thoughts per day.[69] Over the course of a month, that would be about 200,000 thoughts. In a year, that would be over 2.3 million thoughts. If we are stuck with repetitive negative thoughts floating around in our heads, the sheer number of times would constitute reinforcement of the negative thoughts. Thoughts like, "I am ugly," "I am stupid," and "I *always* fail," can be damaging to our sense of self. In fact, I think that one negative thought is more powerful than multiple positive thoughts. A core part of cognitive behavioral therapy is based on this concept since negative core beliefs often generate negative behaviors.

R℞ 5.1 The Thought Ladder and Action Roof Exercise: Try for Yourself
Prescription

1. Refer to Figure 5.2 for an example of using the thought ladder and action roof exercise.
2. Identify a current negative thought you are having. This will be on the bottom rung of the ladder.
3. Set a goal by identifying a thought you would like to have instead. This *goal thought* will be on the top rung of the ladder and will be what you work up to in this Rx.
4. Identify an intermediate thought to work your way up to the goal.
5. Write down ways you can encourage yourself to believe in these intermediate thoughts.
6. Identify another thought that moves you closer to your goal thought.
7. Continue the process of identifying intermediate thoughts that move you closer to your goal thought. This may take 2-10 rungs.
8. Manage your bodily responses. Refer to Figure 4.2 Grounding Techniques. Other relaxation and stress management techniques will be discussed in Chapter 13.
9. Identify ways to take action toward your more positive goal thought.

How do we reset this and replace these negative thoughts with positive ones? One way is by using the Reflect and *Restack* Cycle in Figure 3.2, going through our feelings and thoughts, and arriving at a different lens and solution. Another approach would be one often used by therapists, called the thought ladder exercise. In Figure 5.2, an example of using the Thought Ladder and Action Roof Exercise is displayed. This exercise helps drill down into our thinking by focusing on a negative thought, such as "I hate what my body looks like." By working up the rungs of the ladder, we move through different positive thoughts and ultimately take an action when we reach the roof.

After reviewing Figure 5.2, please try it for yourself with Rx 5.1. Revise your thoughts as many times as you need until you come up with the most positive statement you can. The thought ladder tool helps with cognitive restructuring and resultant behavioral action.

FIGURE 5.2 AN EXAMPLE OF THE THOUGHT LADDER AND ACTION ROOF EXERCISE

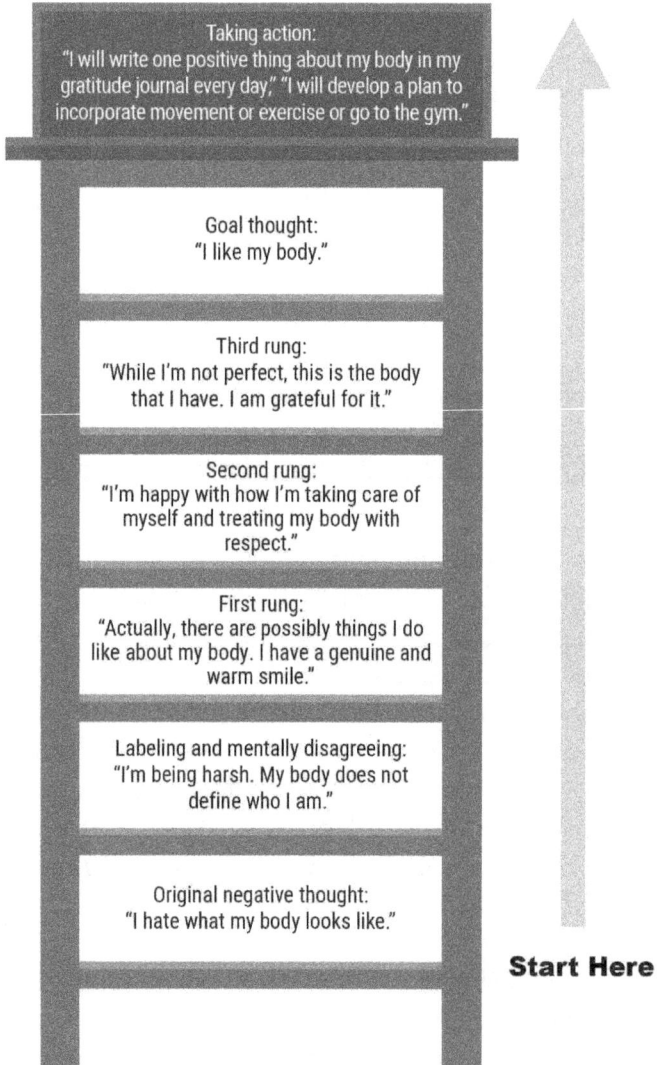

Taking action:
"I will write one positive thing about my body in my gratitude journal every day," "I will develop a plan to incorporate movement or exercise or go to the gym."

Goal thought:
"I like my body."

Third rung:
"While I'm not perfect, this is the body that I have. I am grateful for it."

Second rung:
"I'm happy with how I'm taking care of myself and treating my body with respect."

First rung:
"Actually, there are possibly things I do like about my body. I have a genuine and warm smile."

Labeling and mentally disagreeing:
"I'm being harsh. My body does not define who I am."

Original negative thought:
"I hate what my body looks like."

Start Here

Cognitive Health in Children

When we consider cognitive health concerns, we usually think of dementia in older adults. But, children can also suffer from cognitive issues. Some examples include delayed speech or difficulty speaking, as well as difficulty learning at the appropriate level for one's age, or problems with communication or interacting with others. Lifestyle interventions can be beneficial for children of concern, and many have thrived with the proper interventions. We will discuss these interventions in detail in Chapters 10 through 15.

We also know that a woman's health before and during pregnancy can predispose children to numerous disorders.[70] Multiple studies have revealed that a pregnant woman's exposure to stress and her food choices affect a child's learning and cognitive development years later. The child's cognitive health is important for women to keep in mind during pregnancy.[71,72]

Cognitive Disorders in Adults: Dementia

One in 10 people over the age of 65 suffers from dementia.

Dementia is not one single disease, but includes multiple diseases such as Alzheimer's disease, vascular dementia, and Lewy body dementia.[73-75] *Mild cognitive impairment* is a subtle form of cognitive dysfunction that occurs prior to dementia. It's an early stage of memory loss or other cognitive abilities such as language ·or visual/ spatial perceptions. Over 15% of people with mild cognitive impairment will go on to develop Alzheimer's or another dementia within two years. Over 30% will develop Alzheimer's within five years. Mild cognitive impairment is reversible. Therefore, prevention is still possible during the earlier stages in many individuals.

Cognitive Health in Older Adults

While the cognitive health science for older adults is still evolving, one thing is clear—through modifying our lifestyle, we can potentially lower our risk of developing dementia. In fact, lifestyle interventions may even help with prevention and treatment once cognitive impairment has developed. While the pillars of lifestyle psychiatry are covered in detail in subsequent chapters, because of their significance, we will briefly touch on the pillars to outline cognitive health in older adults here. These foundational lifestyle psychiatry pillars include restorative sleep, nutrition, physical activity, connectedness, stress management, and substance use harm reduction.[76]

Restorative Sleep in Older Adults

Older adults often experience sleep difficulties. This is especially true for older adults who struggle with sleep apnea, particularly in those diagnosed with dementia. Therefore, it may be beneficial to incorporate the sleep hygiene and relaxation techniques suggested in Rx 11.2 and Rx 11.3 in Chapter 11: Restorative Sleep. Overall, emerging research shows cognitive behavioral therapy for insomnia (CBT-I) can aid those with sleep difficulties.[77] CBT-I is a modified form of CBT that uses specific protocols to address the root causes of an individual's insomnia.

Nutrition in Older Adults

Nutrition has been shown to have a significant effect on cognition, through multiple interactions with genetics and the systems in our body and our brain. The diet that has the most potential to, according to research-based evidence, prevent and potentially slow down the progression of dementia is called the MIND diet, an acronym for Mediterranean-DASH Intervention for Neurodegenerative Delay.[78] The MIND diet involves minimizing red meat and ultra-processed foods while increasing green leafy vegetables, berries, whole grains, beans, and healthy fats, such as nuts.

Physical Activity in Older Adults

Cognition is positively affected by exercise. In those with established Alzheimer's dementia, both cardio and strength training are associated with decreased risk of death, as well as reductions in brain dysfunction in the early stages of dementia.[79] Additionally, aerobic exercise has been linked to the release of BDNF and other neurotrophic factors that are implicated in slowing down cellular aging in the brain.[79]

Connectedness in Older Adults

Connecting socially with others plays a big part in dementia risk. Those who suffer from loneliness have a higher incidence of early death as older adults. Loneliness and having a purpose in life have been noted to lead to worsening cognition in older adults by increasing stress, thereby causing inflammation.[18] Even in younger adults, social connectivity is an important element to consider in preventing dementia in later life.[80] All the more reason to get out there and enjoy our time with others —our brains will thank us.

Stress Management in Older Adults

Inflammation occurs when we have higher levels of cortisol due to stress. Increased stress is associated with elevated levels of pro-inflammatory molecules. Chronic inflammation can lead to multiple disorders, such as cancer, diabetes, depression, and anxiety, all of which are risk factors for dementia.[81]

Substance Use Risk Reduction in Older Adults

Drinking more than 14 drinks per week increases the risk of dementia.[82,83] While many scientists argue both sides, the research is unclear whether small amounts of alcohol can actually be protective against dementia.[84,85] Heavy alcohol use can lead to nutritional deficiencies, especially in vitamin B1, also known as thiamine. Early-stage thiamine deficiency can be hard to detect, but can ultimately lead to weight loss, poor memory, fatigue, confusion, and muscle weakness. Over time, someone with thiamine deficiency might develop an enlarged heart and subsequently, dementia. Wernicke's encephalopathy, also caused by thiamine deficiency, is an acute reversible disease of the nervous system, characterized by a triad of symptoms: confusion, difficulty walking (also known as ataxia), and eye abnormalities.[86] Prolonged thiamine deficiency can lead to an irreversible dementia called Korsakoff syndrome, with damage to nerve cells and the brain.[87]

Wrapping It Up

In our busy lives, we often put little thought into what a feeling *is*, what a thought *is*, and what our behaviors *are*. It can be very powerful to intentionally tease out the differences and nuances of each. In this chapter, we have seen just how connected these constructs are. By decreasing our cognitive distortions and negative thought loops, we may be able to *Restack* some of our mental blocks. The Thought Ladder and Action Roof exercise in Rx 5.1 can be used in multiple scenarios as we continue to move toward a more positive and healthier mental and emotional state. Indeed, it would be a missed opportunity to not put all our understanding into action—that's what the behavioral aspect of this chapter suggests.

We are more than just our emotions, cognition, behavior, and sensations. We possess individual personality traits that inform our ability to live the life we want. When someone does something quirky, we often say, "Oh, that's just her!" But are quirks and traits so finite and fixed? As we are growing and developing through the process of self-help, can we also change our responses to situations by *Restack*-ing our personality traits? Let's explore this question next.

Chapter 6: Personality Traits

How do your friends and family describe you? Do they say you are kind? Funny? Helpful?

Many of us feel comfortable with self-help books focusing on habits. It's easy to hear from an expert to examine *this* or tweak *that* in order to make lifelong changes. For many people, this approach works. But what if it doesn't?

What if you're not able to accomplish the goals you have set for yourself just by changing your habits? What components are missing? Often, we feel like failures because while the best-selling book is great, and we really liked it, we're still back where we started, even after trying to change our habits. This chapter and this book are about going deeper than habits.

Yes, changing habits is important. But, for me, as a psychiatrist, it's like asking a 1-year-old to learn how to ride a bike before they know how to stand or walk. Yes, a 1-year-old can learn how to ride a bike, but it may not be the most enduring strategy for success, unless they have the previous foundational pieces in place. The pieces I'm referring to are not actually skills, but include emotions and cognitive elements we discussed in previous chapters—we are now adding personality traits to the mix. Reading this chapter and working through the Rx's will require courage and an honest inventory of ourselves, but it is so worth it.

The Five Major Personality Traits

What words do you use to describe someone's personality traits?

In the field of psychology, the five core personality traits have been described as **N**euroticism, **E**xtraversion, **O**penness to experience, **A**greeableness, and **C**onscientiousness.[88] The acronym OCEAN or

CANOE is often used to remember them. Research has shown these five personality traits, along with their related changes in emotional adjustment, help define who we are as humans.[80-92]

In the previous two chapters, we explored emotions and cognition and how they affect our behavior. We also discussed interventions that may be needed to make long-lasting changes to achieve the habits we want. While those two chapters bring together two important pieces of the puzzle, the third major piece is personality traits. Without addressing our personality traits, we may feel unsuccessful in the emotional and cognitive work we do. To further the conversation, multiple research studies have found that aspects of our personalities, as described in these five major traits, could be associated with our physical health.[93,94] This means those of us with certain personality traits may be at risk for specific *health* conditions.

In Rx 6.1, there are nine questions to help you create an honest inventory of your personality traits. While I chose nine questions for this inventory, those who are interested can look up the longer inventory of personality traits that is referenced on my website www.giamerlo.com, called the Big Five factor.[95] To be clear, this chapter is about personality *traits* not our personalities.

In psychiatry, diagnosable personality *disorders* appear to be present in about 10% of the population.[96] That is, upon evaluation from a psychiatrist, 1 in 10 people will have a diagnosable personality disorder. People suffering from personality disorders may have a difficult time relating to others and maintaining relationships, thereby impairing their personal and work quality of life. They struggle to understand emotions and often are impulsive.

In this chapter, the focus is not on these diagnosable personality disorders, but on personality traits, which 100% of the population have. We all have personality traits–they are normal. In this chapter, we will focus on the pain and suffering some unwanted personality traits can cause and their associations with behavior and diseases.

R̶X 6.1 Honest Inventory of Your Personality Traits
Prescription

Ask 1-2 people who know you well to give you an honest assessment of your personality traits. This can be friends, family, or even yourself. Examples of questions to ask are:

1. Do I worry a lot?
2. Am I social or shy?
3. Am I comfortable with trying new things?
4. Do I trust others?
5. Am I organized?
6. Am I easy to get along with?
7. Do I prefer staying home and "chilling," or do I like being "out and about"?
8. Do I give without expecting others to give back?
9. Do I have good self-control?

Habits versus Personality Traits

In *Atomic Habits,* James Clear proposes that making slight changes in our habits can achieve big results.[97] I wholeheartedly agree that we can achieve explosive results with even the most incremental changes. In *Restack*, I expand the initial concept presented by James Clear to include "atomic" changes in many areas–not just habits– personality traits being one of them. Changes in our personality traits can make a huge difference and lead to better outcomes in our health and our relationships.

Many of us have read self-help books and benefited from the techniques introduced, but many of us have read these books and were unable to make these changes to our habits stick. Why did that happen? Many of my patients who have read multiple self-help books come to me feeling discouraged and demoralized. "How is it possible?" my patients ask me. "I am smart and capable but still unable to nip this in the bud?" *Restack* intentionally includes solutions that help with habits, but also delves deeper into mental blocks. In fact, every chapter in *Restack* expands the conversation for those of us who have not found benefit in self-help books—it's possible that there is more to understand and work on than incremental changes to our habits.

Working at the margins of these issues is sometimes enough to change a person's life. For a time, my social outlets and community engagement only existed through dating. Because I was a single parent with a demanding work schedule, I felt I had to choose between dating or developing a robust social network with my precious spare time. The path forward for me was to prioritize the latter—to find a community of people who allowed me to have positive rewards and fun experiences not dependent on romantic relationships that could be fleeting. I decided I needed to build a community of support that would be a constant throughout the ups and downs of dating. To facilitate that, I joined a Unitarian Universalist church and enrolled my daughter in the Sunday School, which taught lessons from all the major religions. Unitarian Universalists welcome people from all religious backgrounds, including Catholics, Protestants, atheists, and agnostics. It was just one morning a week, but the slight change was so needed for my isolated self.

Personality Traits and Well-Being

The wellness movement is about addressing everyday health for everyone. In contrast, well-being includes wellness and adds a few other deeper elements, such as supporting our potential psychiatric symptoms and the personality traits that don't serve us. With well-being as the goal, the conversation we have with ourselves must be different. Well-being encompasses *Restack*-ing our resilient, well-adjusted self and incorporating these elements as we continue to develop a more rounded, honest, deep, grounded exploration of who we are and who we want to become. Some of us can do this through the self-help techniques presented in this book, and others will need the support of therapists and medication.

For those of you who may be triggered by these discussions, please practice self-care in approaching this chapter. If you find yourself overwhelmed, please move on. Or stop and use grounding exercises (see Figure 4.2) before gently continuing with the book.

Personality Trait #1: Neuroticism

Neuroticism can be simply defined as excessive worry and becoming easily upset, tense, and nervous. Neuroticism is a tendency to have ups and downs in our mood, multiple times during the day caused by seemingly small inconveniences. This is different from the mood fluctuations seen in depression, a mood disorder, or diagnosed personality disorders, which can be confusing at times.

People suffering with mood disorders have *sustained* periods of ups and downs in mood in addition to other symptoms. For example, for a diagnosis of depression you need a two-week period of depressed or sad moods. Neuroticism can predispose people to depression and anxiety, which are further correlated with increased mortality.[98-100] Not only is neuroticism important in depression and anxiety, but for those of us struggling with unhealthy eating behaviors, the anxiety associated with the eating behaviors often needs to be addressed first.

The difference between a neuroticism personality trait and some personality disorders, such as *borderline personality disorder* (BPD), is also important to note. Individuals suffering with BPD not only experience up and down fluctuations in their mood, but also other symptoms such as impulsive behaviors, intense but unstable relationships, and chronic feelings of emptiness.

Overall, while we can see neuroticism manifest in many disorders, it is not a diagnosis but a personality trait. And, all humans have personality traits.

A Case of Neuroticism: My Experience

I am one big neurotic human being, so I have many stories that make excellent examples!

When I was 25 years old, I was a single parent with an infant. Dating and meeting people was high on my priority list, but I worried about my body and wanted it to be as close to "perfect" as possible, the way it was pre-pregnancy. I felt excessively nervous about being seen naked with my cesarean section scar. Everybody has baggage. But unlike most 25-year-olds my baggage included a car-seat and a stroller. A little too heavy for most guys that age, don't you think?

I fell into a loop of telling about 70% of my dates, the first time I met them, that I had a baby, which turned many of them off. The other 30% of the time I never mentioned I had a baby until about two months into dating, which also caused some shock and brought on a lot of questions. This was the 1980s, and I found that most men my age had little understanding of or desire to relate to my experience. In those pre-Internet days, we did not have the abundance of information available that we have now. But beyond that, I didn't want to have to shift a fun, casual conversation between two young people to something intense or serious. They were in their mid-20s after all, what did they know about babies?

How was I supposed to talk to these men about my child and my life situation?

This entire process made me feel pathetic and easily upset while highlighting my neuroticism. I ended up feeling very tense around men and ultimately became discouraged about the entire prospect of dating.

Among other things, as discussed before, I began focusing on my weight and body image.

This short example describes my innate neurotic tendencies that were brought out by my life issues. Rx 6.2 can help you identify your tendencies to be neurotic. Answer the questions presented with "yes" or "no." The more times you answer "yes," the higher your degree of neuroticism.

Body Self-Love Towards a Human-Positive Movement

For me, I just couldn't find the balance. I would go back and forth between watching my diet and letting it go to manage the anxiety I felt.

A current empowering body-positive cultural narrative encourages us to accept our body as it is right now. That movement is extremely important in helping address the excessive worry (neuroticism) that is tied to aberrant eating behaviors like compulsive over/undereating. So, it's great to call out neuroticism for what it is—an unhealthy personality trait akin to a continuous loop in our brain driving us to focus on the way we look.

However, this body-positive movement eventually needs to evolve by adding another step:

I love my body the way it is, and I also love myself enough to want to be physically healthier.

Self-love and a positive mindset can go hand in hand. How about adding to the conversation a *human-positive movement* to become the best version of ourselves physically and mentally? Rx 6.3 focuses on sitting with your worries and encourages you to identify and develop a process to quell anxiety by using grounding techniques. The Rx also includes activities to help tolerate worrisome thoughts with distinctions between those focusing on internal practices we can perform that affect our internal state, versus external practices that help ease the worry.

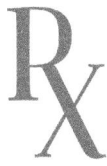

R⚕X 6.2 Assessing Your Neuroticism
Prescription

1. Do you tend to be moody and easily upset?
2. Do you get nervous easily?
3. Do you worry a lot?
4. Do you often feel tense?
5. Do you have difficulties with handling stress?
6. Do you have trouble remaining calm in tense situations?

Note: If you think you should have a formal diagnosis of anxiety or depression, please read Chapter 16 Beyond Self-Help.

Science of Neuroticism

Recent research has examined those of us who tend to worry excessively. The research noted that neuroticism may be helpful for successful aging as increased focus on health through worry leads to better health outcomes and resilience.[98]

On the other hand, another study showed neuroticism can be associated with an increased risk of heart disease and metabolic disorders, like diabetes.[99] Neuroticism is also related to people struggling with being overweight and obese.[100] I strongly believe there is a way we can address the health risks associated with these conditions without shaming our body. Instead, we can treat ourselves with gentleness and kindness, in a way that takes into consideration concepts mentioned in the last few chapters and the social determinants of health, which are discussed in Chapter 8.

R̶X̶ 6.3 Sitting with Your Worries
Prescription

1. Identify three things that make you feel tense or worry you.
2. Choose one of these three things to focus on today.
3. Note the amount of tension or worry you experience on a scale from 1-10 (10 being the most).
4. Use one of the following activities to sit with your worries or nervous feelings. There is no right or wrong activity. These are some examples, but there are many others — choose one that works for you!
   a. **Internally focused activities**:
      i. Mindfulness
      ii. Deep breathing
      iii. Box breathing
      iv. Meditation
      v. Visualization
      vi. Progressive muscle relaxation
      vii. Going on a mindful walk
   b. **Externally focused activities**:
      i. Writing down your worries and feelings
      ii. Journaling
      iii. Drawing, painting, writing stories, dancing, music, and other creative activities
5. If your worries get excessive, use the grounding techniques in Figure 4.2.

Personality Trait #2: Extraversion

Extraversion describes a complex interaction between ourselves and the external world. Extraverts usually have a high desire to be sociable, often seek excitement, and have high activity levels. The opposite of extraversion is introversion, describing those who appear to be reserved, but are not unhappy or shy.[101] In practical terms, introverts tend to look inward. After introverts spend time in a social setting, they may feel the need to spend time alone to recharge or recenter. On the other hand, an extravert is described as a "people person" who derives energy from being around people and external stimulation.[102] Some people may be *ambiverts*, where they have a balance between both features of an extravert and introvert.

Use Rx 6.4 to assess your extraversion. Answer the questions with "yes" or "no." The more times you answer "yes," the higher you score on the extraversion trait.

R̶X 6.4 Assessing Your Extraversion
Prescription

1. Do you tend to be full of energy?
2. Would you describe yourself as enthusiastic?
3. Do you find yourself talkative in most group situations?
4. Would you describe yourself as outgoing?
5. Have you ever been described as a social butterfly?
6. Do people describe you as assertive?
7. After spending an entire day with people, do you feel energized?
   Or, do you need time for yourself to recharge?

A Case of Extraversion: My Experience of "I-Didn't-Know-What-I-Didn't-Know"

Growing up, I always thought of myself as an extravert, but I didn't have the skills to effectively socialize. That was due in part to my being raised in a traditional immigrant family and because English was not my first language. Extraverts can be shy as well—these two states are not mutually exclusive.

As a young mother, in addition to my neuroticism about dating and my body, I worried a lot about keeping my child safe. I had just enough knowledge and experience with psychiatry and the often-not-too-kind world to prevent me from trusting someone else to be alone with my child.

Part of this fear was likely linked to the memories of my abusive marriage, but to an extent, this fear was healthy and warranted. The scary data on the number of stepfathers sexually abusing their stepdaughters hit me like a ton of bricks.[103] I worried obsessively and felt I couldn't add that trauma to my sweet daughter's life. I didn't trust myself enough to protect her from men since I hadn't adequately healed myself. How could I?

I knew that *I-didn't-know-what-I-didn't-know* about the parts of me that led me to marry an abusive man and stay with him for five years. I was determined to figure that out (and am still working on it!) before exposing my daughter to my neurosis.

As a result, I became very focused on my work and began a path of limiting socializing and making friends. To be fair, it wasn't just fear that held me back. I also didn't have the time for a social life—I was a single mother physician after all. Between supporting my daughter's school activities, taking care of my patients, engaging in therapy, and continuing to learn medicine as a lifelong learner, there just wasn't enough time in the day to socialize.

It's interesting how our external day-to-day life affects our personality traits. I believe I behaved more as an introvert because of the realities of my life, though there was still an extravert deep inside of me screaming to get out.

Connectedness Is Both an Internal and External Process

In April 2023, the U.S. Surgeon General released a statement calling loneliness in the U.S. an "epidemic."[104] Isolation is linked to heart disease, hypertension, diabetes, and numerous other conditions.

Connectedness is considered one of the pillars of lifestyle psychiatry and thus has Chapter 14 dedicated to it. We will discuss connectedness briefly in this chapter because introverted people may socially isolate and, thus, not enjoy many of the benefits of connectedness.

In my case, throughout my 20s and 30s, I stagnated in my emotional intelligence because I was spending so much time inside my head and wasn't engaging much socially.

Increasing our connectedness can involve both internal and external processes. The internal process of connectedness amplifies parts of our personality traits. An example of the internal process is the art of feeling gratitude, which is described in more detail in Chapter 13: Stress Management. Feeling gratitude functions as a way to develop stronger and healthier connections with the outside world. That is, gratitude allows us to internally set ourselves up to proceed to the external process of connectedness.

The external process of connectedness involves our interactions with those around us and our actions in the world. This can be achieved through communication, i.e. having conversations, knowing how to use small talk, conveying empathy and respect, managing our tone and eye contact, and using clear speech. Without first engaging in the internal process of gratitude or other feeling states, it may be difficult to sustain healthy communication in our daily life.

Practice the exercises in Rx 6.5 to improve your communication, thereby enhancing your potential for achieving connectedness often.

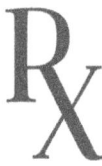

R℞ 6.5 Exercises to Improve Your Communication
Prescription

1. **Active listening:** During two conversations next week, set a silent timer for 2 minutes (or 5 minutes if you're courageous), and listen to someone without interrupting. Take mental notes of what the other person is saying. After they finish speaking, repeat back to them what you heard to make sure you understood them correctly.

2. **Receiving feedback:** Ask someone you trust for feedback. Feedback can be from something you did together, a project, a task, your cooking, or anything that requires honesty and good communication. Listen in a non-defensive way. Thank them for their honesty.

3. **Giving feedback:** With the same person you received feedback from step #2, ask if they're willing to receive feedback from you. The feedback should lead with the positive, be supportive and specific, identify areas for improvement, and involve a conversation between the two of you after you deliver the feedback.

4. **Apologizing:** Apologize to someone you trust and are close to. Use all the elements of an apology, which are acknowledging the error, explaining what happened, expressing remorse, and suggesting a reparation. Try this first with a simple apology for something like knocking over the salt shaker. Apologies involve very complex interactions and may be difficult and stressful. It's important not to get defensive and to take responsibility.

Dopamine and Extraversion

Even as someone who was naturally shy, I was an extravert (remember, they are not mutually exclusive, and they are not the same thing!) and I missed having friends. Extraverts are sensitive to dopamine and rely upon the dopamine reward system for pleasure.[105] When my extraverted traits were suppressed, and I was not able to socialize and get the reward of dopamine, I had to find balance through the activities listed in Rx 6.6. These dopamine-regulating activities are discussed in further detail in Part D of the book.

R℞ 6.6 Dopamine-Regulating Activities
Prescription

Make a habit of daily practices that enhance your happiness and pleasure. There are many dopamine-regulating activities discussed in this book that correspond to physical activity, nutrition, stress reduction, connectedness, and sleep. A few examples include:
1. Daily gratitude exercises or other meditative practices
2. Listening to music
3. Getting more natural sunlight
4. Trying new hobbies
5. Dancing or other fun movements

Personality Trait #3: Openness to Experience

Openness to experience means being comfortable with the unknown and willing to try new things. While agreeing to skydive is an example of openness, this trait is more than just willingness to perform risky/thrilling activities. The expanded definition includes a willingness to consider ideas and experiences which are unlike our past experiences. It also includes being available to get out of our comfort zone of what we believe to be true. Openness happens when someone brings up an idea or thought, and we can think or say, "Oh, that sounds interesting. Let me try it." We may acknowledge some discomfort with the idea, but we are still willing to give it a try.

For example, if your friend loves playing an instrument, or wants you to attend their church service, or recommends you read a book outside your normal interest, or try Ethiopian food for the first time, do you take a stab at it with a positive attitude, or do you say, "No, I could never do that"? This trait is about opening a space within our comfort zone to allow for a new experience instead of dismissing an opportunity upfront.

In addition, the stories I describe in this book of embracing aesthetics—art, nature, and beauty—are also examples of welcoming openness to experience.

The Science of Openness to Experience

Scientists have highlighted that openness to experience can be connected to health outcomes.[106] Multiple studies have found those with greater openness to new experiences have a decreased risk of early death from all causes, also called *all-cause mortality*.[107,108] Interestingly, they are also protected from obesity and heart disease.[109-112]

A Case of Closed-mindedness: My Experience

In my life, one of the major changes I had to undergo for my health was developing a willingness to date people who weren't ethnically Indian. I married into a conservative Hindu Brahmin family. That's all I knew. He was the first man I lived with and had sex with (after we were married, mind you!), and it formed the basis of my identity. At first, I was not willing to think outside that boundary. I had a firm belief that I had to be with an Indian man, ideally a conservative Brahmin man. But the dating pool for me in that category was practically nonexistent once I was divorced with a child.

Because I was unwilling to imagine other realities, I was also attracting men who were unwilling to imagine other realities. On a basic level, I was just looking for someone who would replace my ex, so everything could go back to the way it had been. This led to a cascade of problems around my eating behaviors. I was trying to control my body and eating, thinking I could make myself attractive to these men when I should have been looking beyond them.

Once I opened myself up to other possible dating realities and allowed myself to think that my path and my life could be different, I considered other templates—not necessarily getting married, and maybe meeting people with other lived experiences. I became less obsessive in my eating behaviors and less concerned with controlling my environment. This process required me to clearly differentiate what my values were and identify the areas where I was willing to be open to new experiences.

What Is Your Value System?

Our personal values help determine what is most important to us.[113] Our values usually are what drive us every day. They can include prioritizing friends, spending time with family, working to increase our income, focusing on our careers, seeking personal growth, engaging in romantic partnerships, having fun, expressing our concerns about our environment, improving our health, volunteering and being altruistic, practicing religion, and engaging in creative ventures.

Rx 6.7 asks you to take an inventory of your value system. Sometimes our tightly held beliefs and values may keep us trapped in our unhealthy coping behaviors. Having values is vital, but it is also helpful to differentiate what our true values are from what are just habits, which may or may not be serving us well. To grow and develop, we have to mourn and accept the loss of value systems that do not benefit us anymore.

Personality Trait #4: Agreeableness

Agreeableness means wanting to be in harmony with others, having the capacity to give without getting back (altruism), and trusting the world and the external environment.[114] A person's agreeableness, like most personality traits, is on a spectrum. While most of the personality traits discussed in this chapter operate inside us, agreeableness is primarily an interpersonal trait focusing on socialization and connectedness. We discussed connectedness as it relates to personality trait #2, extraversion, above, and will discuss connectedness more extensively in Chapter 14. However, connectedness is a key component of agreeableness, which leads to our ability to be altruistic, work well with others, and feel a sense of harmony.[114]

R℞ 6.7 *Restack* Your Value System
Prescription

1. **Write** down some of your values.
2. **Identify** value systems that are beneficial, as well as value systems that may not be serving you well anymore.
    a. For example, a less beneficial value system may be staying up all night playing video games instead of getting enough sleep or spending time with loved ones.
3. **Label** the value system that may not be serving you anymore as an *undesired* value system.
    a. For example, choosing to spend too much time playing video games instead of practicing a healthy lifestyle is an undesired value system.
4. **Acknowledge** what the undesired value system means for your identity.
    a. For example, someone might say, "I'm a top-ranking gamer."
5. **Recognize** how the undesired value system offers structure to your life as well as other benefits it may provide.
    a. For example, someone might say, "I have a great time connecting with my gaming buddies online."
6. **Restack** the benefits of the undesired value system so you can seek them elsewhere. Are there ways you could increase socialization and find a community? Are there other places where you could develop a healthy identity, get positive affirmations, and find a sense of meaning and purpose?
    a. For example, someone might say, "The social connection I feel online with my gaming buddies will no longer be as strong. But I will be able to form closer relationships with my friends from school. I will also be able to get enough sleep, which should help me concentrate better and perform better on my tests."

Unless we have trust in ourselves, it's hard to trust another person. In order to be altruistic, cooperative, and generous, most individuals need to feel trust on four levels: the self, an individual, our community, and a higher power. Trust in a higher power may be of a religious or spiritual nature and may not apply to everyone. But the four levels of trust are not necessarily linear. Some people may have issues trusting other individuals, but are able to trust a community, a group, or a society. In my case, I trusted my work colleagues, and I trusted my religious group. Individuals may trust whatever tribe they are a part of. Though agreeableness is a personality trait, in certain situations, our ability to trust may be derailed by our external environment—for example, through experiencing trauma, being taken advantage of, or feeling betrayed. These external factors may cause hiccups in our ability to trust on one or more levels—or do the opposite. For example, after trauma some people may indiscriminately trust everyone around them, thereby potentially continuing the cycle of trauma.

The ultimate trust is trusting that the world is inherently good and that it will take care of us. Though trending downward in the U.S., over 75% of people around the globe believe in a religious order.[115] And while 75% is a resounding majority, even more people are spiritually inclined. With recent global issues like the pandemic, political unrest, and worries about climate change, many people have stopped trusting. Some are struggling to see the positive in the world. We are living in confusing times. The lack of trust currently felt by many makes it difficult to know who we are and our purpose in life.

A Case of Agreeableness and Trauma: My Experience

When I was young, being married to an abusive man changed me in many ways. Over time, I became so accustomed to saying yes to everything he wanted so as to not anger him or create waves. This sort of *hyper*-flexibility, being cooperative and forgiving his ever-present abuse broadened and deepened my ability to be agreeable. But was it healthy? Or was I a victim who got lost in the downward spiral of this sado-masochistic sort of marriage? Indeed, at night I had trouble sleeping, I was fearful, I had a startle response that was exaggerated and I was, for a lack of a better word, mousy.

I bring up this case to highlight the point that though some personality traits may serve us and be healthy, they may have been developed or heightened due to prior difficult lived experiences. My wanting not to make waves in my relationship was so extreme that I altered my sense of reality in order to cause less arguments, in a sense, the way Ingrid Bergman's character did in the 1944 film, *Gaslight*. Through my marriage, my agreeableness factor went up exponentially because I was trying to keep the relationship together. Though the marriage was horrible, I sharpened my ability to be cooperative, kind, generous, and more agreeable. I would have to work through my trust and the trauma, but the bonus was I knew how to connect in a flexible way. I experienced *post-traumatic growth*, which refers to how a reclamation of a traumatic lived experience can help a person grow in a positive way. And, spoiler alert, I didn't have to go through the "psychosis" Ingrid Bergman endured in the film.

Use Rx 6.8 to assess your agreeableness. Answer the questions with "yes" or "no." The more times you answer "yes," the higher you rate on the agreeableness trait.

Viktor Frankl's *Man's Search for Meaning*

Many of us struggle to maintain a positive view of the world and trust society, communities, and individuals. We struggle for good reason. The ability to forgive, trust, and be generous and warm with others requires us to see the world in a positive light. Several notable authors have helped me develop traits of trusting and forgiving others, the foremost of whom is Viktor Frankl.

In my second year of psychiatric residency, a few of my co-residents and I formed a book club with a senior psychoanalyst on faculty. We read Viktor Frankl's *Man's Search for Meaning*, which none of us had read previously.[116] From his inhumane treatment during the Holocaust, Frankl developed a theory called "logotherapy," which is built on several key principles—the foremost being that our primary motivational force in life is to find meaning—and holds that no matter how bad our circumstances, our freedom to hold on to our purpose in life informs and gives meaning to our suffering. He believed those who survived Auschwitz understood that this basic freedom couldn't be taken from them, even while they lay naked, body-to-body in the camp's sheds.

R̷X 6.8 Assessing Your Agreeableness
Prescription

1. Do you tend to forgive others?
2. Do you consider yourself kind, considerate, and trusting of most people?
3. Do you enjoy cooperating with others and working in a team to reach a shared goal?
4. Do you tend to see the best in others?
5. Do you find yourself being generous and helping others, without expecting anything in return?
6. Do you avoid quarreling whenever possible?
7. Do you feel that you warmly engage with others?

Positive Psychology

Frankl's ideas for how to treat patients and how to envision a positive state of the world have many parallels to the discipline of *positive psychology*, a term first coined by Abraham Maslow in 1954.[117] The field was further expanded to the scientific study of human flourishing applied for optimal experiences and positive functioning in 1988 by Martin Seligman.[118] Liana Lianov, founder and president of the Global Positive Health Institute, sees the field of positive psychology further expanding to positive health, where thriving goes beyond addressing traditional risk factors and facilitates individuals becoming their best selves in the face of illness.[119]Both Frankl's theories and those of positive psychology ultimately encourage agreeableness through benevolent and altruistic behavior.

Foster Children

When I worked in a community clinic in Philadelphia, I interacted with many foster children who came from homes where they were sexually and physically abused. One of the hardest concepts to understand was the fact that foster children often had a habit of stealing from others. These were usually small things, like chalk from the classroom or a bobby pin from the teacher's hair. I've known patients who would have a special place to store all the items they stole from others.

Because of the abuse the foster children had experienced in their lives, these small objects were necessary psychological tokens for them. Taking these objects helped the children feel mastery by allowing them to unconsciously equalize the wrongs done to them.

Much of the therapy with these children involved building up their *ego strength* and a sense of themselves. We would use *play therapy* to gradually provide the child with a positive adult interaction they could internalize as loving, kind, and non-abandoning. Over time, they would feel more whole inside. As the children became more trusting of the people in their universe and their abandonment wounds eased, we watched the stealing behaviors often decrease as well.

Feeling that the world will take care of us, and that we can also trust the world, are both necessary for developing the trait of agreeableness.

The Journey of Healing and Developing Altruism

I was fortunate to have had a childhood devoid of the extremes of trauma—I was not physically or sexually abused as a child. But, the trauma I endured during my marriage had cut to the bone of my internal sense of safety. Therefore, I felt I could relate in some way to these foster children. Even though my trauma happened when I was technically an adult, I had manifested a few behaviors similar to those of the foster children. As an example, I borrowed two books from my supervisors and never returned them. I understand this act sounds tame, but it was something I did very intentionally and was not keeping with my normal behavior. It emerged from a compulsion to take, and I am horrified when I reflect back on it.

To this day, I still have those books, and they remind me of that compulsion—that need to fill my emotional cup. I now often find myself giving books to others, as if the act might not just undo the theft, but also all my human failings. I have evolved to become a more trusting person, and I now thrill in the process of giving to others. While I consider myself a lifelong learner and lifelong *Restack*-er, and as such, a work in progress, I hope my healing journey can serve as hope for others who may be facing similar struggles.

The Science of Agreeableness

Having a low level of agreeableness is related to what we often call a "type A personality." Many people with this trait struggle with a lot of anger, which is considered a risk factor for heart disease.[120,121] Recent research looking beyond the Big Five personality traits notes subdimensions of agreeableness that include cynical hostility, which was seen as low agreeableness.[122] This level of agreeableness, which is a combination of hostility with submissiveness, has been associated with an increased risk of early death.[123]

Engaging in altruistic or compassionate actions activates the pleasure centers in our brains that bring us fulfillment and happiness. When we're able to live in a sustained state of altruism—learning to let go, sharing our resources, opening ourselves to others—we feel more happiness. These traits may point to a changed dynamic of giving and receiving with joy. It's a state we often lose sight of in modern culture, where we're arguably taught to take, taught to need, and taught to measure and count our money and resources more often than we're taught to give without a thought.

Personality Trait #5: Conscientiousness

Conscientiousness is a personality trait encompassing self-control, organization, planning, and other frontal lobe activities. Even if we have addressed all the other traits in this chapter, if we don't have self-control, we often won't be able to maintain a healthy relationship with ourselves and practice healthy lifestyle behaviors. Arguably, even if we cultivate the right tools, change our mindset, and other aspects of who we are, without the brain structures to organize our lives and exert self-control, the work won't be effective. Developing tools such as regulating our emotions, grounding ourselves, and breaking our thought loops are all valuable skills, but conscientiousness is required to give us direction.

For many of the patients I've seen over the years—even those without trauma—small incremental changes in conscientiousness can make a significant difference. I've found an eclectic approach is helpful, through providing tools to help with planning and self-control, releasing the burdens of emotional baggage, and *sometimes* incorporating medication and external support.

For some who are just not able to exercise on their own, creating appointments with an exercise buddy or joining an accountability group might be necessary. Many people are embarrassed about the need for accountability. These individuals are often intelligent and capable in many areas of their lives, but they just can't follow through with physical activity—they often find it difficult to accept this mental block. Though it's an external way to create organization, if we continue to use accountability long enough, the benefits of mastering our task will ultimately outweigh the embarrassment we might feel about needing external support.

Use Rx 6.9 to assess your conscientiousness. Answer the questions with "yes" or "no." The more times you answer "yes," the higher your conscientiousness trait.

R
X

6.9 Assessing Your Conscientiousness

Prescription

1. Do you consider yourself organized?
2. Are you attentive to detail and do a thorough job with your tasks?
3. Are you overall efficient with your tasks?
4. Do you make plans and generally follow through with them?
5. Would others describe you as reliable?
6. Do you usually persevere until a task is finished?

The Science of Conscientiousness

Conscientious people are known to follow through with their plans and stick with them long-term. This leads to general health benefits that have been studied by numerous researchers. High conscientiousness is associated with a lower overall risk of mortality.[93,94] Interestingly, high conscientiousness is also associated with a decreased body mass index and obesity risk. There are also lower levels of an inflammatory marker called C-reactive protein, often abbreviated as CRP.[124] The protective mechanism leading to low mortality may be mediated by an inflammatory marker called IL-6.[125] While the science behind conscientiousness and our body's immune responses is continuing to unfold, the current research suggests that being conscientious has multiple benefits for our overall health.[126-128]

Putting It All Together With the Pillars of Lifestyle Psychiatry

Table 6.1 summarizes the concepts discussed in the chapter.[129-151] This table is organized by the six lifestyle psychiatry pillars which is the first column. The second column lists numerous behaviors or processes we may be struggling with like repetitive thoughts, insomnia, etc. In order to read this table, you can start with the behavior you want to learn about in column two. Then look at the third column to see the individual personality traits associated with these behaviors.

As an example, are you someone who eats unhealthy foods? If yes, this is listed as a behavior in the second column. Now, look at the corresponding third column. The third column lists the individual personality traits that research notes are associated with this behavior. In this example, the personality traits we often find in someone who eats unhealthy foods include high neuroticism, low conscientiousness, low agreeableness, and low openness. Armed with this information, we can go back through this chapter and study ways we can improve these personality traits, thereby trying to improve the behavior of eating unhealthy foods. This is an important step in the process of *Restack*-ing ourselves!

Lifestyle Pillar	Behavior or Process	Personality Trait
Nutrition	Eating unhealthful foods	High neuroticism
		Low conscientiousness
		Low agreeableness (antagonism)
		Low openness
Physical activity	Engaging in physical activity	Low neuroticism
		High conscientiousness
		High extraversion
		High openness
Stress management	Interpersonal conflict	High neuroticism
	Daily hassles	High neuroticism
	Repetitive thoughts and worries (generalized anxiety disorder and depression)	High neuroticism
	Fewer stressors caused by situations within your control, e.g. planning	High conscientiousness
Connectedness	General poor health outcomes	Low agreeableness (antagonism)
		High conscientiousness
Sleep	Increased disease risk	High sleep time variability and duration variability
	Decreased clearance of metabolic waste from the brain	Low overall sleep duration
	Improved sleep duration	High agreeableness (antagonism)
	Greater sleep deficiency (the discrepancy between duration and self-reported sleep need)	High neuroticism
		Low extraversion
	Preference for early morning waking	High conscientiousness
		Low openness

Table 6.1 What the Science Says About Personality Traits[129-151]

Table 6.1 What the Science Says About Personality Traits (continued)		
	Insomnia	High neuroticism
		Low openness
		Low conscientiousness
Substance use	Current smoking status	High neuroticism
		High extraversion
		Low conscientiousness
	Smoking initiation	High extraversion
		Low conscientiousness
	Higher potential for smoking relapse	High neuroticism
		High extraversion
	Transition from moderate to heavy alcohol use	High extraversion
		Low conscientiousness
	Transition from moderate alcohol use to abstinence	Low extraversion
		High agreeableness
		Low openness
	Alcohol involvement	High neuroticism
		Low agreeableness
		Low conscientiousness

Conclusion

We cannot change what we have not named.

Changing the key personality traits I've described above seems like an enormous task to address. But it is important to understand how science and research explain the traits. While the research around personality

128

traits and behaviors is still emerging, I hope that some of you may find this chapter valuable and actionable. These personality traits are not just personality quirks, there is a connection between our brain and the traits. If you have unhealthy behaviors or processes, you can refer to Table 6.1 and try to adjust parts of your personality traits as a strategy to release some of the mental blocks and *Restack* yourself.

My assessment of my own personality traits has evolved over time, and my sense is you will note the same in yourself. I hope sharing my stories helps others who may be struggling in similar ways or who know others who are also struggling. My point with this chapter is to help others understand we are connected as humans, with our vulnerabilities, quirks, experiences, and our traumas. I am forever inspired by the courage that writing down and verbalizing our experiences provides. It not only helps us identify who we are at a given point in time, but also allows us the freedom to evolve. We cannot change what we have not yet named– awareness needs to happen before change.

Part C: External Barriers

Chapter 7: Work-Related Burnout

Though it's been used since the 1970s, burnout is a word we hear now more than ever.[152,153]

Burnout is a term that is used frequently in conversation to represent extreme stress in our personal and professional lives. For the purposes of this chapter, I will be using the medical definition of burnout which necessarily is in response to burdens in the workplace. To be sure, with this definition, work-related burnout can bleed into our personal lives. For those of us experiencing extreme stress and burnout related to either non-work related situations or work-related situations, you may find this chapter most useful when read in addition to Chapter 13.

Definition of Burnout in the U.S. and Globally

Rapid advancements in technology have led to an "always-on" culture, blurring the boundaries between work and personal life as well as increasing work demands. The COVID-19 pandemic and its aftermath have added significant stress and uncertainty to people's lives, disrupting routines, increasing isolation, and heightening anxieties.[152,154] Economic pressures, job insecurities, and the continuous pursuit of productivity have created a high-stress environment in the workplace. Additionally, the constant exposure to social media and the rise of "comparison culture" has fueled feelings of inadequacy and contributed to the epidemic of burnout. We often find ourselves with less and less time to adequately practice self-care, which further exacerbates the issue.

These complex interplays of societal, economic, and technological factors have led to a widespread burnout epidemic, highlighting the urgent need for comprehensive approaches to address and alleviate this modern-day challenge.[152]

In the U.S., burnout is often defined as a state of chronic physical and emotional exhaustion, typically resulting from prolonged exposure to work-related stressors—it is characterized by feelings of cynicism, detachment, and a reduced sense of personal accomplishment.[155] Burnout is particularly common in high-pressure work environments where employees experience overwhelming demands and limited resources to cope with them. This lack of resources and support is very different from the way some other countries approach burnout. In Sweden and the Netherlands, for example, burnout is a diagnosable condition, and therefore, insurance covers the available treatments and people can receive disability benefits.[156,157] Insurance payments for treatment and disability benefits for burnout are unheard of in the U.S. and most other countries!

Use the questions in Rx 7.1 to assess your level of burnout.[158] The more times you answer "yes," the higher your burnout.

R̶x̶ 7.1 Are You Burned Out?[158]
Prescription

1. I feel ineffective in my job.
2. I don't feel I am making a positive impact through the work I do.
3. I feel worn out and tired from my work.
4. I feel increased mental distance from my job.
5. I find myself cynical towards people at work.
6. I'm struggling to care for people at work and instead see them more like checkboxes on a to-do list.

Who Gets Burned Out?

Burnout affects workers across all industries, but I mostly use examples of physician burnout when I talk about this problem because this is my field, and I have been able to study (and experience) it firsthand.

In the United States, during the pandemic data showed over 60% of physicians experience burnout, a statistic that holds true across many other professions.[159] There are enormous structural consequences to untreated burnout in healthcare. For example, over 30% of nurses are expected to leave their jobs within the next five years.[160] So why does this matter? It costs millions of dollars to retrain new health professionals to fill the vacated jobs, so burnout also becomes an economic burden to our community.

On an individual level, burnout can lead to more serious mental health issues—an increased risk of anxiety and depression, for example.[161] If we don't put more resources toward addressing the burnout epidemic in the U.S., we're going to end up with widespread economic and health problems. The questions are: Are we already there as a country? And how are we doing globally?

A Case of Burnout

Ross is a 42-year-old manager of a Fortune 500 company, where he has been with the same company since graduating high school. He has always been a hard worker and notably well-liked by fellow employees, new hires, and upper management. In 2016, following a merger by his company, he was kept on, but was expected to absorb the workload of two laid-off employees. Ross found this taxing but felt honored management had confidence in his abilities. During COVID-19, the company faced a financial downturn, and in another series of layoffs, Ross had to fold another team's worth of work into his already stretched responsibilities.

Ross came to me for treatment because he was showing up later and later to work, was feeling increasingly negative and cynical, and would snap at his kids at home. He no longer enjoyed his job, felt he was failing as a manager since he didn't have the pulse of the employees anymore, and kept getting swamped by emails. Ross felt he had lost control of his work environment and the ability to keep up with the day-to-day decisions he had to make. He had to cut down on his volunteer tutoring of kids in the neighborhood and found himself in front of the computer all day long, with limited to no social interactions. Ross's work started to feel mundane and more about keeping the company afloat and cutting back much-needed resources from employees.

He was showing the classic three symptoms of burnout I mentioned earlier: cynicism, detachment, and a reduced sense of accomplishment. Ross denied, and there was no evidence of, thoughts of hurting himself or others, problems with sleep, or other risky behaviors or thoughts. For Ross, the solution was not to give him an antidepressant medication and tell him, "You're depressed, see you in couple of months for a follow-up." While there is some overlap in symptoms of depressive disorders and burnout, there are distinct differences. If Ross had displayed risky symptoms or met the criteria for major depressive disorder, of course, medication would have been the first line of treatment followed by psychotherapy and lifestyle interventions as appropriate.

The remedy for burnout symptoms is not one-size-fits-all. While burnout is a common result for many people experiencing overwhelm at work, the solution often involves a process we will cover later in this chapter. Burnout reduces an individual's ability to make decisions because the person is often constantly assigning blame to themselves. Ross's treatment involved empowering him to make decisions, whether that meant staying in the job or leaving.

As is true for many people in Ross's situation, sometimes knowing we have choices, as well as the power to make them, can help ease the stress of a situation.

Another Case of Burnout: My Experience

I went straight into medical school from high school without a clear understanding of what it meant to be a physician. I wanted to please my parents and had the typical "physician-to-be grades." Decades later, when I was a dean advising premedical students, their struggles reminded me of my own. These stellar, motivated, straight-A students didn't know what the profession was really like.

Seeing my struggle repeated in these students helped me stop blaming individuals for the problems in some educational institutions. A lack of understanding of the responsibilities of a physician is not an omission by family members, but often a problem with the educational system, which doesn't give students enough realistic exposure to the work of being a physician. *Grey's Anatomy* and other popular portrayals that glorify the life of a physician don't help either.

Many physicians went into medicine thinking they were going to heal people but didn't really have a thorough understanding of the day-to-day grind, particularly the time required for paperwork and administrative tasks. Later, I went on to develop a college course that provides premedical students with enough exposure to clinical medicine to make sure they have the right aptitude, attitude, and ultimately desire once they knew the good, bad, and ugly of medicine. Being a physician means spending your days for the rest of your career with sick people who are suffering. The curriculum was immortalized into an academic book for physicians called *Principles of Medical Professionalism*[162] that I published with Oxford University Press (indeed, writing books is my coping strategy—we can argue whether it's healthy or not. I have that argument with myself all the time).

While I now have a firm hold on my professional identity, that wasn't always the case.

At the age of 34, I was a single parent, deeply in debt, and becoming disillusioned with clinical medicine. While fantasizing about leaving the profession, I had just completed my residency, but I had to stay in the job until I paid off my loans. I wasn't qualified to work in any other jobs that would get rid of my hundreds of thousands of dollars of debt. So, I continued as a full-time mother and psychiatrist, working in the community and private practice settings for the next 10 years. But as soon as my daughter left home for college in 2006 and my responsibilities lessened, I started to feel the full weight of my burnout. There was no joy left in the profession for me, and I showed all the classical signs of burnout, as outlined in Rx 7.1. I'm certain many other working adults felt the same, but few conversations mentioned burnout in the early 2000s. Because I didn't understand what was happening, I thought getting out of medicine was the solution. I got an MBA, left the field of medicine, and took a job on Wall Street as a financial adviser. Was this a healthy change or an avoidance tactic?

My Detour as a Financial Adviser

Looking back, things that were hazy back then are now crystal clear.

My detour as a financial adviser was one of intense learning, but was not aligned with my core personality and definitely not my emotional and cognitive strengths. Indeed, in a way, I still felt like a physician even though I was working in finance. I was taking care of people's money instead of their mental health, but I had the same mindset of working as hard as I could for the benefit of others. I was still acting like a healer but offering financial care.

After a few years, I had enough distance from my burnout to realize I am a physician at my core. I have the mental makeup of a physician. I just

138

had the wrong job, and I needed to get off the *hedonic treadmill* and only work in positions I really love. I had to acknowledge to myself that healthcare is corporatized and about making money for the stakeholders, and thus often dysfunctional. Despite that, I felt I could still do a lot of good for patients. My dissatisfaction with medicine was not about the profession itself, but more a rejection of the workhorse environment.

So, I went back to medicine.

Finding My Emotional Fuel

I knew I wasn't going to be able to solve the structural problems within the healthcare industry, so I refocused on what I wanted out of the job: a healthy professional relationship with patients. I found a company that didn't necessarily have all the prestige of the shiny, high-powered jobs I may have wanted before, but it provided more support for its physicians and allowed me to focus on what was important to me. I had more time for my life outside of work. Instead of having financial metrics on my mind, I was able to find joy in the small wins with my patients, like when they thanked me for a session or when one of my interventions worked for them. Having one or two of these wins a week kept me fueled.

Physicians in the U.S. Are Employees, Not Decision-Makers

While modern medicine has evolved to become more evidence-based and secular, the historical ties between medicine and religion have produced an expectation that physicians treat their job as a calling and put patients before themselves.[163] Multiple mandates and core competency training for physicians involve medical professionalism, which insists on this exact mandate. Patients come before the clinician.

Such an ideal runs counter to the current corporatization of healthcare, where physicians are often hourly employees with little control or influence over the structure of clinics or hospitals.[164] Physicians have little control over the number of minutes they're allotted during their day with each patient or the number of patients they see, but are still often dinged in online reviews for long wait times. Burnout often occurs for physicians because of the gap between expectations and reality. They come into the profession thinking of it as a high calling of service and healing, but the job is no longer really about that.

Consequences of Burnout

As you can imagine, if you extrapolate from the two cases presented in this chapter—my case and Ross's case of burnout—burnout has a significant impact on well-being and the quality of life of workers. This leads to job dissatisfaction and retention issues. Exhausted and emotionally depleted employees may experience reduced empathy and engagement, leading to job errors and reduced productivity in the workplace. Burnout also increases workers' risk of developing mental health disorders and suicidal thoughts.

In healthcare specifically, burnout can deter individuals from pursuing full-time medical careers or lead physicians, nurses, and others to leave the profession prematurely. This contributes to a shortage of healthcare providers, especially in certain medical specialties and underserved areas. Burnout can result in higher healthcare costs due to increased medical errors, patient readmissions, and decreased productivity. Strategies to combat burnout include promoting time away from work to rejuvenate, implementing support programs, improving work conditions, and fostering a respectful culture prioritizing the well-being of healthcare professionals.[165]

These strategies to address burnout can be adapted and applied to all disciplines, not just medicine.

Strategies for Burnout Prevention

How can we prevent burnout?

The National Academy of Medicine, an organization composed of all the major medical specialties, has been working to solve the systemic issues in the workplace.[166] Multiple structural interventions in healthcare are beginning to appear including addressing the burden of electronic health records and how that is interfering with workload and connectedness to patients. In addition, interventions and education to address burnout in physicians include programs such as the *Steps Forward* program.[167] While these structural changes are ongoing, we are not powerless as individuals. We can take steps to shield and empower ourselves in these environments.

Burnout can be addressed before it happens or after it occurs. In the United States, burnout is not considered a diagnosis, like diabetes, depression, and anxiety. That's important for treatment considerations since we need a formal diagnosis for insurance to cover the treatment or intervention.

When available, interventions can occur at any point in the progression of burnout, including preventing burnout before it occurs, decreasing the worsening of burnout once it occurs, and providing resources once burnout has taken full hold. These strategies are all called prevention techniques by medical professionals, though they can also be "treatments." We can think of burnout prevention in four stages: primordial, primary, secondary, and tertiary prevention as shown in Figure 7.1.[168]

Primordial prevention includes strategies to avoid risk factors before any symptoms appear. This is a matter of general well-being and maintaining health through lifestyle factors such as restorative sleep, healthy relationships, etc. These will be discussed in detail in Chapters 10 through 15.

Primary prevention occurs after symptoms appear. This kind of prevention involves normalizing the struggle, processing the emotions of work (see Chapter 4), talking about the moral distress, promoting self-efficacy, addressing unmet needs, decreasing isolation, targeting organizational issues (not just system organization but changing our individual response to the organization), and addressing individual personality traits that may be contributing to the problem. These strategies are presented throughout this book (especially Chapter 6 on personality traits) and aim to empower people to thrive in less-than-ideal environments.

Secondary prevention occurs when the burnout has already taken hold. This kind of prevention is about reducing the severity of symptoms. Mostly, this means coping with and managing stress, in addition to using all the tools mentioned in the previous two types of preventions. Each stage of prevention builds on the previous stages. This is described in detail in Chapter 13 on stress management.

Tertiary prevention is about connecting people with outside resources, beyond what they can do for themselves by managing their lifestyle and their relationship to work. Some of these resources might be providing referrals to employee assistance programs, psychiatric evaluations, medical treatment for symptoms, suicide prevention resources, and addiction support groups.

Burnout Interventions

In the previous section on strategies for burnout prevention, multiple interventions are described. Some consistent themes run through this four-stage model of burnout prevention. Two of these are lifestyle and personality interventions.

FIGURE 7.1 THE FOUR-STAGE MODEL OF BURNOUT PREVENTION [168]

Individual-focused burnout risk reduction strategies can target primordial, primary, secondary, and tertiary prevention.

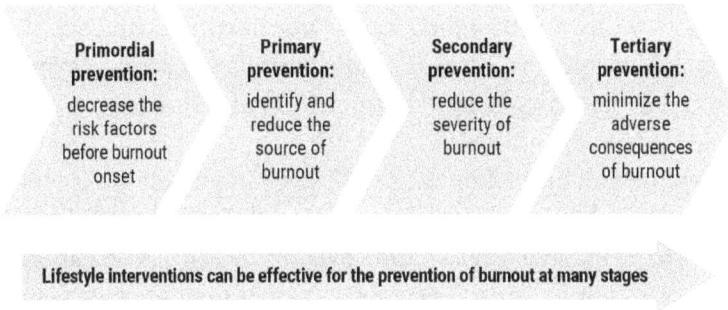

Primordial prevention: decrease the risk factors before burnout onset

Primary prevention: identify and reduce the source of burnout

Secondary prevention: reduce the severity of burnout

Tertiary prevention: minimize the adverse consequences of burnout

Lifestyle interventions can be effective for the prevention of burnout at many stages

Adapted with permission from Merlo G, Rippe J. Physician Burnout: A Lifestyle Medicine Perspective. Am J Lifestyle Med. 2020 Dec 29;15(2):153.

Lifestyle and Diet

Burnout is not just a matter of workplace stress and exhaustion. It impacts and is impacted by a range of lifestyle factors—our sleep quality, physical activity, social connectivity, etc. which are described in Chapters 10 through 15.

Burnout and Eating Behaviors

The correlation between burnout and unhealthy eating behaviors, for example, is significant, as chronic stress and emotional exhaustion can lead individuals to seek comfort and relief through food choices that are often unhealthy.[169] When experiencing burnout, people may turn to sugary, high-fat, and ultra-processed foods as a coping mechanism to alleviate stress and provide temporary emotional comfort. This emotional eating can lead to weight gain, nutrient deficiencies, and disruptions in the body's metabolism, further exacerbating feelings of fatigue and low energy.

Additionally, burnout can disrupt normal eating patterns, leading to irregular mealtimes and skipping meals, which can negatively impact overall nutritional intake. The cycle of burnout and unhealthy eating behaviors can create a detrimental loop. Poor nutrition can contribute to decreased resilience to stress and worsen burnout symptoms, perpetuating a vicious cycle that hampers overall well-being.

Addressing burnout and adopting healthier eating habits are essential for breaking this cycle and promoting a more balanced and sustainable approach to managing stress and overall health. A balanced and nutritious diet rich in fruits, vegetables, whole grains, plant sources of proteins, and healthy fats can support stress management, mental clarity, and general resilience. This can play a vital role in preventing and mitigating burnout's impact on physical and mental health. With everyone being so busy, a solution that could work is to look at options in your area for weekly food delivery programs that emphasize healthy and easy meals, or to subscribe to a box program that delivers fruit and vegetables to your door. Many of my patients have benefited from these delivery programs. While some of my patients use these temporarily as a bridge to healthier eating, some use these long-term. For more information, refer to Chapter 10: Nutrition. Further resources are available on my website www.giamerlo.com.

Personality and Burnout

When we are young, part of the process of developing our psyche is the back-and-forth process of making mistakes and learning from them. This helps us learn over time that we will survive despite our flaws, and we are ultimately good enough. Many of us weren't given the opportunity to learn from our childhood errors, either because we were always striving to be perfect (and succeeded!) or more commonly, didn't have enough practice in reflecting (see Figure 3.2 Reflect and *Restack* Cycle). Learning how to fail *well* is a skill we all need to develop. It took me a long time to learn this lesson, and it's one that I keep needing to relearn.

When I left the medical profession, on some level it felt like I was a major failure. But ultimately, it helped loosen my need for perfection, which improved my mental and physical health. It also allowed me to redefine myself, not take myself too seriously, and develop emotional fortitude.

Much of my perfectionism had come from a desire for external validation. I wanted to please the medical system, and I wanted to be 100% for every patient every time. Every minute of every hour with every patient, I listened intently. I had to make sure I heard everything. When I left healthcare and worked in finance, I would overhear people around the office say things like, "Oh, well, I forgot to do such-and-such. Sorry." Within many jobs in finance, these mistakes are often accepted as part of doing business. The team works together to problem-solve, and the environment feels less toxic. Whereas in medicine, errors are costly on many levels—at the least we get a slap on the wrist, but most often, we get formally written up. How can we all individually ensure we treat ourselves with compassion for our imperfections, in a system that may not be as forgiving?

Take-Home Message

While in this chapter I focused on the example closest to me, which is the burnout among healthcare providers, these scenarios are very similar to other professions. As with Ross in the first case example, work environments contribute to burnout and constitute external blocks. Initially, Ross's block wasn't about him. But over time, because his external environment (the company he worked for) did not change (because he needed a job in order to make money, like most of us do) and the mergers and increased workload happened so fast, his burnout crept in and became an internal problem for him. So even though the cause was something external (work), he was left with an internal struggle that transferred to other areas of his life (his family).

For those of us who have the opportunity to and are able to change jobs or careers, that's often a good option. But in my case, jumping to another career was ill-informed. I should have focused on learning how to cope with and manage what was triggering me in my external environment. Ultimately, I think we all need to give ourselves the opportunity to slow down enough and use the strategies presented in Table 7.1 to reduce our

Table 7.1 Individual Strategies to Reduce Burnout[170]	
Strategy	**Interventions**
Self-reflection	- Use the Reflect and *Restack* Cycle (Figure 3.2)
Changing job partners	- Working less - Taking more regular breaks
Developing coping skills	- Time management (Chapter 13: Stress Management)
Building social connectivity	- Colleagues, supervisors, and family that target employee's relationship with work (Chapter 14: Connectedness)
Fostering good health	- Lifestyle interventions in Chapters 10-15, such as healthy eating and exercise
Stress reduction techniques	- Cognitive behavioral techniques - Relaxation - Mindfulness - Self-efficacy-based interventions - Chapter 13: Stress Management
Tweaking personality traits	- Perfectionism - Neuroticism (Chapter 6: Personality Traits)
If you have psychiatric symptoms	- Getting a psychiatric evaluation (Chapter 16: Beyond Self-Help)

state of burnout. Burnout is a very real problem and there is a high rate of substance use in people suffering from burnout. It affects a sizable percentage of the population and is a significant external barrier to improving our collective health. Whether your burnout is work-related or general burnout, using the tools expressed in Chapter 13 on stress management may be helpful.

When you're ready, turn your attention to Rx 7.2 "Reflecting on Your Burnout." This Rx encourages you to identify the stage you're in using Figure 7.1, and then to systematically review Table 7.1 for strategies to help provide relief from burnout.[170] Make sure to get outside assistance if you are overwhelmed or have severe symptoms. You might also refer to Chapter 16: Beyond Self-Help for more information.

℞ 7.2 Reflecting on Your Burnout
Prescription

1. Review the left column of Table 7.1 Individual Strategies to Reduce Burnout. Reflect on the strategies you want to work on.
2. Consider employing the interventions referenced in the right column of Table 7.1.
3. Make sure to seek outside resources if you are overwhelmed or experience symptoms that are severe. See Chapter 16: Beyond Self-Help.

So, burnout is one external block we addressed in this chapter. In the next chapter, we address other external barriers related to health and the environment. It's clear that the environment we live in is less than perfect. But let's consider what we can do for ourselves despite this limitation.

Chapter 8: Our Environment and Health

If we don't have our basic survival needs met, all other approaches to well-being are a waste of time. This is the basic tenet of our existence as humans.

In the last few chapters, we discussed internal mental blocks that can impede us from living the life we want, such as trauma, a lack of emotion regulation, our thoughts and cognitive distortions, our personality traits, and our internal reactions to our work environments. These blocks are all very real and, at times, extremely debilitating.

Our external physical environment also has a powerful impact on our mental health. Blocks created by our environment may include a lack of healthy food options, climate change, toxins in our foods, an unstable housing situation, and other social determinants of health. Maintaining positive mental health involves addressing these external barriers as well as our internal states and responses.

Though many of us are safe, well-fed, and housing secure, we may know or care about others who struggle with one or more of these elements. In fact, even if we don't know others who struggle, understanding how the environment impacts humans is a necessity for an evolved, well-functioning society. In this chapter, we will delve into these topics with the lens of deepening our understanding of ourselves and our fellow humans.

Please note that much of the information in this book references U.S. data because that is where I reside, but these concepts can be extrapolated to many other countries' populations.

We are all in this together.

Our Current State of Mental Health Treatment:
How Did We Get Here?

People forced to live with housing insecurity is a public health travesty.

In the 1950s, changes in federal legislation to close chronic mental health facilities pushed the burden of treating mental health to the community, such as in outpatient settings.[171-173] These chronic mental health facilities allowed patients to stay for years and sometimes decades. Now, in the U.S., in-patient stays are measured in days and those struggling with chronic mental illness are often discharged without a roof over their head. Shifting the treatment to the community initially seemed like an effective way to provide the least-restrictive care for patients. Unfortunately, with the funding for community centers dwindling, those who would have received treatment in community outpatient settings for chronic conditions, such as schizophrenia, no longer had access to the resources. These resources were often lifesaving and included safe housing, medication for mental stabilization, educational resources and support for family members, and social workers to help them navigate the complex healthcare system.

These patients continue to fall through the cracks even now. Multiple studies have shown that low-income communities experience a higher incidence of mental illness.[174-176] This is partly because they have less access to resources for prevention, and partly because of the considerable strain of the challenging realities of their situation. Of course, it's difficult to generalize an individual's situation within any demographic. I don't want to stigmatize low-income communities by linking poverty with mental illness. I mean for this chapter to highlight the environmental factors contributing to mental illness and to elevate the conversation around them.

My Experiences with Community and Private Practice Psychiatry

When I worked as a child psychiatrist in inner-city Philadelphia, many of the children I saw came from low-income homes. I loved working in this clinic because it provided me with a much-needed perspective since my private practice was on the other end of the socioeconomic spectrum. While the mental health needs of the two population extremes somewhat overlapped, their needs were generally very different. Overall, the suffering in both populations was very real. The inner-city work didn't pay a lot, but it kept me balanced and in touch with the larger community. I often found myself filled with rage to see the disparities between the two demographics.

In many families, corporal (physical) punishment, for example, was accepted, and I was tasked with identifying where it crossed the line into a reportable offense.[177] The World Health Organization notes that globally 60% of children ages 2 to 14 will regularly be physically hit.[178] If a caretaker spanks a child without leaving a mark, is that reportable to child protective services? What if the caretaker used a rod? A belt? Do I need to examine every child for physical marks at each visit? Keeping my personal bias about right and wrong was necessary as I began to understand the differing uses of discipline. Having this dual-demographic practice early in my career expanded my knowledge of psychiatry by leaps and bounds.

The result was that I became emotionally receptive and flexible in my thinking as a physician and with my treatment methodologies. Over time, I recognized similar patterns of discipline between the two seemingly disparate groups. Some of these patterns could have been upsetting and problematic for me. As a mandated reporter, I (and all healthcare providers) am obligated to report evidence of or knowledge of abuse. But I was able to shift to an approach of creating a stable space where the families could feel safe talking about what they were doing at home. They needed to trust that I would help them and not pass judgment. Often the line between my obligations to help and to protect was very fine. However, I learned to listen better, leave my biases at the door, and understand that there are many ways to raise children depending on the family circumstances. Looking back now, I am almost embarrassed to have been paid for the education these working experiences afforded me and the tremendous professional growth they inspired.

A Case of Food Insecurity

One of my patients, a 9-year-old named Benjamin, came in to be evaluated for ADHD after his second school suspension. According to his teacher, Benjamin was unable to sit still, would walk around the classroom, and would randomly get into fistfights with other kids. Upon meeting with him alone and after engaging with him in conversation and play in my office (play is often used to evaluate and then treat young children), I found Benjamin shy, curious, and eager to please. If I said something he didn't like, he jumped up and became activated but was easily able to shift back into calmness.

He reported the only place he ate food was at school because he "didn't like eating breakfast" and was "too busy to eat dinner at home." I often had a bowl of healthy snacks in my office for just these occasions, which I unfortunately was seeing increasingly with my patients. I offered to have a snack together while we continued our session, and I saw his eyes light up with unabashed eagerness—he was hungry. I asked if his mom and siblings ate at home, and he said, "No, we just don't do that."

He hesitated and then looked up at me for a moment and asked, "Does my mom get one?"

I said, "Sure."

He said, "And my brother?"

Before I could answer, Benjamin jumped out of his seat, chose snacks for his mother and brother, and he joyously took the snacks out to them in the waiting room. He then came back and chose one for himself.

As we talked, he described the bullies at school who would try to take his lunch from him. Getting suspended meant no food, he said, but letting them take his lunch also meant no food. His logic was sound and thoughtful.

Though Benjamin met the criteria for ADHD, I suspected he also needed social and economic support, not just a medication known to decrease appetite. The number of children globally on medication for ADHD has increased enormously—approximately 1 out of 16 children are taking it.[179] Many children absolutely need the medication for ADHD given that it is a brain disorder, but up to one-third of the children do not respond to the medication. I suspect some of the non-responders could be due to environmental factors or other aspects of their symptoms that were missed when they were diagnosed.[180]

An array of environmental factors in Benjamin's life, beyond what I've described here, were impacting his mental health and his behavior. For example, I learned about the "juice" his parents bought at the store, which was just sugar, water, and food coloring. This "juice" was popular among the inner-city Philadelphia community, as it was sold for 10 cents in the neighborhood food markets. I also learned that after he got suspended, his mother would beat him when he got home. His neighborhood had limited parks and limited safe outdoor green spaces like playgrounds. Thankfully, his school still made time for recess and PE, but the only space available was a small parking lot. At home, he didn't play outside because it was known to be too dangerous. He told me that he often heard fights going on in the streets outside his home, and gunshots often appeared in his drawings. The most common entertainment for him was watching television and video games which I have found can contribute to a misdiagnosis of what appears to be ADHD.

On the surface, if one were to just do a checklist on ADHD symptoms, Benjamin would meet almost every criterion.[181] But was ADHD his diagnosis? It was not clear to me at the time, but in most present-day clinics, he would have been diagnosed and started on medications. Taking his social determinants of health, environmental stressors, and food insecurity into consideration, we have a different picture of the interventions he needs. By doing what we can to *Restack* these external blocks in Benjamin's life, we would allow him to reach his potential and thrive. Resources, support for the family, and empathy are the keys here. And maybe medication would be indicated too once his basic needs had been addressed and the picture became clearer.

What Is "Real" Treatment?

The pressure is very high for a psychiatrist to diagnose behavioral symptoms and medicate children, and adults as well, instead of trying to deal with the environmental aspects of our patient's lives. We can't fix many of the environmental problems, and ethically, we aren't allowed to involve ourselves in their lives to that level.

Honestly, I have bent the rules at times.

A Case of Environmental Barriers

Katrina was an 11-year-old enrolled in a novel school-based partial hospitalization program. This program was for children whom the school system identified as "disruptive." In most situations, repeatedly aggressive children would be transferred to a disciplinary school, often one hour away from their home, if not farther. In Katrina's case, she was placed in the program because of her anger issues. She had multiple suspensions from school for fist fighting with her peers and ultimately threw a chair at her fifth-grade teacher.

The children in this school-based program received intensive psychiatric interventions until they could reintegrate back into the classroom. The only requirement from the parents was to attend monthly therapy sessions and, once every six months, to sign a consent form for their children to continue in the program. If they did not sign the consent, the children had to be discharged. For most of these children, being discharged without completing the program meant being expelled from the school and transported daily via bus to the often far away disciplinary school.

On one March morning, Katrina's parents didn't show up to the six-month meeting at 9 am to sign the consent form allowing her to continue with the program. At this juncture in treatment, Katrina was blossoming. She was learning to control her anger, getting better at expressing her sadness about the death of her father, and opening up about all her struggles at home. She often gave us hugs, was gentle and kind to her peers, and had a vibrant loving smile that made my day. When her parents didn't show up, I became nervous. I feared that Katrina might regress back to her old behaviors if we had to discharge her from the program before she was ready.

I found Katrina's address on the intake form and realized her home was just three blocks away. I called her mother, and my heart skipped a beat when she picked up the phone. Mom said she was too tired to come to the meeting. As I was pleading with her to come to the school to sign the form, she hung up. I looked over at my team, and we all had tears in our eyes. We were so close. We knew we could help Katrina if we had more time with her. In a moment of desperation, I picked up my purse and headed toward the door. My team members looked surprised but hopeful. They yelled, "Don't go without us!" We made a house visit.

I knocked on the door, and when Katrina's mom answered, she was all at once embarrassed and grateful. She smiled and asked us to come in. I glanced around the room and took in the surroundings. I immediately noticed a trail of cockroaches traveling from the floor to the ceiling in the living room. Looking up, I saw part of the ceiling was missing. The visual I encountered was similar to one I remembered from the aftermath of tornadoes and hurricanes from my hometown in Louisiana. Part of the ceiling appeared to be in a state of suspended animation, with clothes barely latching onto water-stained tiles destined to land on the living room floor at any minute. Towels and plastics partially covered the hole in the ceiling. I then looked down at the floor on the other side of the living room. Towels and blankets were arranged there like makeshift beds. Katrina had told me she slept in the living room with her family, and I was seeing it now firsthand.

Katrina's mother asked me if I would have a seat, and I had to check my privilege as an image flashed before my eyes of cockroaches crawling into my purse and all over my body. I had never before seen this level of disrepair in a home in the U.S. outside of weather-related emergencies. In fact, the scene was close to my memories of my time in medical school in India when I had treated patients who lived in mud huts with straw roofs. They often didn't have shoes, would use discarded plastics in ingenious ways in their homes—to patch holes in the roof, make umbrellas, toys for the children, and even to make small huts.

I felt so much sadness for Katrina's family and anger at their situation. These thoughts and feelings had all flashed through my head in the few seconds between her question and my answer. I felt a pang of guilt rejecting her hospitality as I replied, "No, thank you, we'll just be here for a minute."

I talked to her about the treatment plan for Katrina and asked her to sign the form, which she did without hesitation. Mom spoke of being tired after having to ration her insulin shots because of some issue at her clinic.

155

She was confused about the next steps for managing her diabetes but was so thankful for our visit.

Our team helped Katrina's mother get connected with more resources for her medical needs. She was assigned a case worker who checked in with her regularly and was given tokens to take the bus to her appointments. And Katrina was able to stay in the program until ultimately being discharged six months later.

The Social Determinants of Health

I tell the story of Katrina because it demonstrates my blocks in understanding the social determinants of health. My apparent lack of education around poverty in the U.S. was displayed in Katrina's case. I bring this up here not to shame myself, but to draw our attention to these pressing issues and help us build compassion for others. How could I really help Katrina if I didn't appreciate her home life and her family's struggles within it?

Social determinants of health, as first described by Dahlgren and Whitehead in 1990, are factors in someone's environment that are nonmedical but play a big part in shaping their health outcomes.[182] These determinants of health include where and how someone lives, their social and economic resources, their daily habits, and the influences in their lives.

Multiple behaviors in families used to get me riled up, and the process of dispelling my internal biases was not a simple, linear one. The two cases I discuss in this chapter are examples. Parents not showing up to their children's psychiatric appointments and children receiving corporal punishment at home were exceedingly infuriating to me. It was easy to blame or vilify parents for the children's issues. I especially became annoyed and heartbroken internally when mothers would show up to the appointments with perfectly done hair and nails, when I knew they were receiving government aid. I had to learn to understand how much these parents were suffering, too. Their focus on self-care, like meticulously attending to grooming their hair and nails, was often one of the only ways they had of finding some joy in the midst of difficult situations. As expected, many of the parents had their own unmet needs because of their high-pressure environment. Who was I to judge from my place of privilege?

After years of getting to know this Philadelphia community better, I began to appreciate how strong the sense of community was. In fact, it was much stronger than I had experienced elsewhere. I wondered if some of this was by necessity—the community often came together to look after the children. In my own life, I had experienced so much shame around being divorced and held strict ideas in my mind about what a family structure looked like. These families often didn't have those structures I thought were required and, and to my amazement and delight, didn't worry about them. Many women had children as teens, and there often was an amalgam of people who contributed to care: the grandparents, the great-grandparents, other relatives, and neighbors. This social connectivity and support helped the children feel safe and loved. I'm eternally indebted to this community for teaching me these valuable lessons.

Unfortunately, outside of this communal support network, the children were often living in a system designed to make them fail.

Moving forward, let's consider just a few of the systemic factors that ultimately contribute to negative physical and mental health outcomes for both caretakers and their children. These include systemic environmental factors like the air we breathe, air quality indexes, heat and mental health, and toxins in the building structures around us.

Systemic Environmental Factors Affecting Our Lives

Over 99% of the global population breathes unclean air. Air pollution causes seven million deaths per year globally, and untold years of poor health.[183]

Our environment has been burdened with toxins, deadly air quality, asbestos in our buildings, pesticides, and pollutants for decades. We could argue about why it has come to a head at this point in time and discuss the polarity these conversations create in the public, but this is beyond the scope of this book. What we know is our physical and mental health is tied to these environmental onslaughts. It is logical, then, that lifestyle changes can help in our efforts to also sustain the environment.

The Health Consequences of the Air We Breathe

We've all heard that ozone is poisoning the planet. But did you know it might be poisoning us, too?

Ozone is symbolized as O_3 and is a gaseous substance with three oxygen atoms. It occurs naturally in the air we breathe but can also be made by man and has detrimental effects on human health.

There are two types of ozone. One is in the stratosphere, which is natural and helps protect the Earth from dangerous ultraviolet (UV) radiation. Ground-level ozone, however, is mostly formed from human activities and consists of volatile organic compounds (VOCs) and nitrogen oxide. Ground-level ozone sources include fossil fuels, chemical and power plants, and automobile emissions.[184]

How is human health affected by ground-level ozone? Our lungs and mucous membranes can become irritated. Chronic exposure to ozone can lead to airway inflammation, difficulty breathing, and early death.[185,186] This is a circular loop with lifestyle issues coming into play. People with chronic lung problems exercise less, and it is known that physical activity is tied to quality of life and mental health.[187] If the quality of our air is poor, then recommending people to go out in nature may not be advisable.[188]

Apart from ground-level ozone, which is invisible and undetected by our senses, particulate matter (such as smoke from fires and dust storms is visible to the naked eye. In the body, particulate matter is associated with an increased prevalence of high blood pressure, obesity, and diabetes.[189,190] During exercise, we breathe faster to bring in more air, which brings in more toxins to our lungs and our bodies. We become at greater risk of heart, lung, and kidney disease.[191]

Air Quality Index

We could argue the quality of the air we breathe is as important as the books we read, the food we eat, and the company we keep.

Local communities provide free resources online to gauge our air quality index (AQI). In the United States, www.AirNow.gov is a website providing regular updates. Globally, the world's air pollution real-time AQI can accessed here www.waqi.info.

The AQI ranges from 0 to 50 (good), 51 to 100 (moderate), 101 to 150 (unhealthy for sensitive groups), 151 to 200 (unhealthy), 201 to 300 (very unhealthy), and 301 and higher (hazardous). Above 300 is considered an emergency affecting everyone living in the area. It is recommended to limit outdoor activity and exposure on the days when or where the AQI is above 100 for people with lung diseases such as asthma, older adults, children and teenagers, and people who are active outdoors. For these sensitive groups, the recommendation is to make outdoor activities shorter and less intense.

In Rx 8.1, please find the air quality index for your local community.

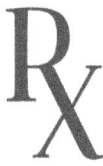

R
X
8.1 Finding Out Your Air Quality Index
Prescription

1. Find the Air Quality Index for your local community. For the U.S., you can go to AirNow.gov, and globally, the website is: https://waqi.info/.
2. Consider limiting exposure to outdoor air on the days when the index is high.
3. Make a list of indoor physical activities on the days you need to limit outdoor air exposure.

Pollution and Mental Health

More research is linking air pollution with worsening mental health, especially depression and suicide risk.[192] The depression associated with air pollution is primarily caused by an abnormally decreased volume of specific regions of the brain, like the prefrontal cortex, hippocampus, and amygdala.[192] In addition, growing air pollution is associated with structural and functional changes in the brain, including increased inflammation and oxidative stress, as well as changes to brain neurotransmitters. Anxiety and depression are the most common mental disorders in the world, and 99% of the world's population does not live within the World Health Organization's definition of safe air.[183] While depression has many causes, it requires us to pause and question how related these two may be, especially as we're seeing worsening mental health around the world.[193-195]

Heat and Mental Health

For every one degree Celsius above 37° Celsius, studies have shown increased health consequences for people with depression.[196-198] For psychiatric conditions in general, heat impacts almost all disorders, including substance use disorders, anxiety, mood disorders, psychotic disorders, self-harm, and childhood behavioral disorders.[199,200] Some of this can be attributed to sleep disruption during warmer nighttime temperatures. During the day, higher temperatures can also act as a stressor that increases irritability.

Research is ongoing to tease out the exact biological cause of how increased heat worsens psychiatric conditions, but we cannot deny the psychological toll it's taking on society.

Climate Anxiety

Climate anxiety has been finding its way into the psychiatric literature as a new concern many people are experiencing.[201] While this was unheard of in the recent past, now researchers are focused on understanding how anxiety around the climate impacts overall mental health. Those of us suffering from climate anxiety describe feelings of a lack of control, worries about safety, and concerns of existential threats related to climate change. Recognizing and naming our feelings around the climate are very important. Consider using Rx 6.3 "Sitting with Your Worries" to help better control the anxiety.

Toxins in Our Built Environment and Our Food

Despite all the enormous benefits we receive by living in a modern society, there are also downsides.

Our built environment basically refers to the human-built aspects of where we live, play, and work, such as our homes, streets, and the community infrastructure. Much of our built environment may contain environmental toxins that can affect our health.

Table 8.1 Common Toxins in Our Environment	
Environmental Toxin	**Effect on Our Health**
Bisphenol A (BPA)	BPA is used to make certain plastics and is known to be an endocrine disruptor (which means they are chemicals that interfere with the normal and natural hormones within our body). BPA exposure causes a dysregulation of estrogen and thyroid hormone, affects our appetites, and is associated with obesity.[202-204]
Lead	Lead is a naturally occurring substance that may be found in soil and certain products (like ceramics and plumbing). Many of us remember the drinking water crisis that occurred in Flint, Michigan due to lead pipes.[205] Lead is also a contaminant in many spices.[206] Lead causes neurotoxicity, and many of these effects are irreversible. Children can have different learning difficulties, whereas in adults, lead may affect the kidneys and elevate the blood pressure.[207]
Radon	Radon is a naturally occurring gas produced by the breakdown of uranium. Radon is a known carcinogen. It is the second leading cause of lung cancer, after smoking.[208]
Phthalates	Phthalates are chemicals that have been used in the processing of plastics and other products. Also an endocrine disruptor, phthalates are associated with obesity, high blood pressure, increased lipid levels, and heart disease.[209]
Arsenic	Arsenic is naturally occurring. Inorganic forms are toxic to humans. Arsenic pesticides and ways to preserve wood techniques are responsible for much of the contamination that enters our food supply. Rice is a big source of arsenic in our food supply.[210] Arsenic is an endocrine disruptor that is associated with type 2 diabetes, increased blood pressure, and cancer.[211]
Mercury	Mercury is naturally occurring. Contaminated shellfish, dental fillings, and rice may also be significant sources of unhealthy mercury in our diet.[212] Mercury leads to neurotoxicity and is associated with high blood pressure and colorectal cancer.[213-217]
Pesticides	Pesticides can be endocrine disruptors and are associated with certain autoimmune disorders (such as Hodgkin's lymphoma), kidney cancer, and liver cancer.[218-220]

Table 8.1 lists some common toxins in our environment and their effects on our health.[202-220] These toxins may be in our built environment, air, or food. While these are listed separately, many have additive (meaning the unwanted effects of the toxins add to one another) or synergistic effects (meaning the effects of the toxins interact in a way that leads to an even greater increase than the sum of their individual effects). Take a moment and reflect on your potential exposure to any of these toxins using Rx 8.2.

℞ 8.2 What Is Your Exposure to Common Environmental Toxins?
Prescription

1. Review Table 8.1 Common Toxins in Our Environment.
2. Take note of the toxins you may be exposed to. Consider different settings you frequent, such as your home, work, neighborhood park, etc.
3. Brainstorm strategies you can employ to limit your exposure as much as possible.

Climate Change

In 2023, the United Nations Climate Change Conference (COP28) elected to make two-thirds of the food served during the conference plant-based for the first time.[221] We will discuss the health importance of whole food, plant-based diets in Chapter 10: Nutrition, but here it's crucial to point out that moving toward a more plant-based overall diet can also significantly influence our planet. By acknowledging the global impact of greenhouse gases and diet, COP28 has made a significant stride forward toward planetary and personal health.[222]

Recent studies have shown that our food supply chain contributes approximately 25% of the world's greenhouse gas emissions.[223] Deforestation and distribution of food products add to this amount significantly, making it closer to 34%.[223]

For example, one kilogram of beef requires 60 kilograms of carbon dioxide equivalents to produce when you include land use, farming, processing, and transportation. Minimizing how many times a week we eat beef can reduce our carbon dioxide equivalent, thereby decreasing greenhouse gas emissions.[223] Moving away from an animal-based diet and increasing plant-based food consumption could reduce our land use and greenhouse gas emissions by significant amounts, impacting the climate change crisis in transformational ways.

To affect planetary health, the changes to our diet don't need to be drastic, but rather mindful of incorporating the consumption of plant-based foods into our daily lives.

Food Deserts

Someone who is parched in a desert takes whatever liquid comes their way.

Food deserts, or areas with limited or no access to fresh fruits and vegetables, are a known problem in many urban communities.[224] Some patients would tell me it takes them two or three bus rides to get to a market with fresh food. Settling for ultra-processed food and fast food just makes more sense for them. Who has extra bus money and two hours to spare to travel? Fast food marketing companies often target these kinds of neighborhoods. If they offer a two-dollar value meal, they know families will line up for it because it's the cheapest thing around. And it's also the easiest way to fill everyone's belly—at the expense of food quality and the effects on our health. We can do better as a society.

164

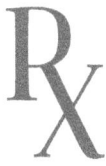

R_X 8.3 Increasing Your Plant-Forward Meals Per Week
Prescription

1. Make a list of the typical meals you eat per week. For example, if you eat three meals each day, that would be 21 meals per week.

2. Note how many animal-based servings you eat per week. Animal-based includes things like meat, chicken, fish, eggs, cheese, and dairy.

3. Consider replacing some of the animal-based servings with whole food, plant-based servings of foods. An example of this would be replacing a pork dinner with meatless rice and beans and a side of vegetables. We will explore this further in Chapter 10: Nutrition.

A Case of NYC Solution Food Changes

Some cities are working on solutions to the food desert phenomenon. In New York City, for example, many of our food banks are adopting a policy of stocking the shelves with 80% fresh fruits and vegetables. In fact, since 2019, NYC administration has been supporting the distribution of one million plant-based meals every month.[225] Nonprofit agencies teaching cooking and providing recipes have also made a substantial impact. Many young parents value how these resources give them confidence and help build a foundation for healthy cooking and eating. The city has instituted Meatless Mondays within all city school systems. All 11 state-run hospitals have defaulted to healthier plant-based menus, though patients can still ask for something different. Now at least patients who have just had a coronary artery bypass aren't being fed unhealthy fried foods and steaks by default. Though some may argue plant-based eating is expensive, plant-based menus are ultimately saving money for the hospital system. Overall, these changes are moving our health in the right direction.

In Rx 8.3, consider possible changes you can make to increase the number of plant-based meals in your diet.

Other Concerns in Communities

Many other factors play into the mental health capacity of each community. These include traumatic life experiences, social exclusion or isolation, unemployment, underemployment (having the education for a higher paying job but not working in one), high-demand/low-control work, childhood abuse or neglect, poor neighborhood conditions such as a lack of community amenities, discrimination, poor access to and lower quality of healthcare and education, and limited social support. Let's start by discussing one of the most gut-wrenching issues of our time, housing insecurity in the U.S.

Housing Insecurity

Housing insecurity is correlated with mental illness in two distinct ways. On one hand, those with mental illness have historically tended to be in the lower economic strata of society, which often means experiencing housing insecurity in urban areas. On the other hand, a majority of the homeless population experiences mental illness. This reality carries multiple burdens, including lack of access to social services without an address on record, high incidences of crime and abuse, and health conditions from living without adequate shelter.

In fact, the single highest population increase recently is of people living in their cars—even among educated individuals. It's been noted that many college students live in their cars, and 1 in 9 college students don't have the funds to afford three meals a day.[226-228] This also impacts what foods these students have access to. Without a fully functional kitchen, they can't cook, store fresh produce, or keep spices to make their food tasty. And, the added strain of housing insecurity is also likely to lead to mental health issues.

166

These kinds of struggles necessarily cause a person stress, which may increase levels of anxiety and depression. Eventually, a breaking point in their ability to cope is reached. While I described a few patients with strong connections to their families or other support systems in this chapter, the situation can be even more challenging when that support doesn't exist.

Compounding Environmental Issues

If someone is struggling financially to put food on the table, and they've been marginalized by the community, that marginalization will not only make it harder to get access to resources but will also erode a person's confidence and self-efficacy. Resorting to using substances or getting involved in crime to meet basic needs constitute failures of our society. For example, what happens if someone is a teenage mom and doesn't have family members who can offer care and support? Often, they may have to drop out of school, and they may only have minimum-wage jobs available to them. These jobs often aren't sufficient to even pay for childcare. It can become an endless cycle. Some of our public school systems in the U.S. have responded with options to offset these issues, such as offering in-school daycare for students who are parents. Still, these measures usually don't solve all the problems of housing or other resources needed to care for a child.

Acknowledging that these environmental factors exist is half the battle because these structural phenomena are frequently beyond our awareness. With our *unconscious bias*, we oftentimes don't even know the right questions to ask. We may have mental blocks to the struggles of the less fortunate in society. In addition, we may have blocks to the environmental health issues we face, such as air quality and societal overreliance on ultra-processed foods. Addressing these blocks and *Restack*-ing them is part of breaking this cycle.

A Global Perspective to Shake Our Thinking

Living in a different country and immersing myself in the culture catalyzed a profound shift in my outlook and appreciation of the world. By listening and doing the research, we can begin to see so much that was once beyond our understanding.

I had been to India numerous times and seen poverty there, but it was still different to see it in the U.S. Growing up in my upper-middle class home in Louisiana, I was shielded from so much. In India, there are stark class separations. The monthly income of the lower labor class is about $60 a month.[229] Basmati rice and other high-priced grains cost about $60 a month to feed a family. Yes, that's right. The cost of a kitchen staple in most homes is the entire monthly budget for a lower-class family. How did they afford to eat? Lower labor class have separate shops selling much lower quality rice for a few dollars per month. These shops also provide clothing and other toiletries that are completely different from what middle- and upper-class Indians buy and use.

While my psychiatric and formal education helped me become more empathic and aware of disparities within the U.S., this Indian experience brought my education to a whole other level. I often wonder if other ugly and pervasive deep disparities and cultural norms existing in the U.S. that I just can't see for what they are. Indeed, my education and need to expand my awareness are never done.

Conclusion

Understanding these environmental factors will then shape the way we engage with ourselves, our families, and our communities. In the next chapter, we'll discuss how the treatment of our mental and physical health can be improved by taking lifestyle factors into account.

While those of us who are compassionate and concerned about our fellow humans understand social determinants of health and inequities within our culture, I would argue we still have blocks and biases. These blocks prevent us from being fully aware of our unconscious biases because the status quo is so embedded into our culture.

For example, when I moved to India for medical school, I had to reexamine what I considered normal in my day-to-day. While I was great at picking up Indian society's biases vis-à-vis disparities in the quality and price of rice in the indigent versus the affluent, I was unsure how to respond when my Indian acquaintances questioned similar biases we have in the U.S. They asked why, in one of the richest countries in the world, are there so many people who can't afford healthcare or are forced to sleep in the streets? Sometimes, it takes looking at our lives from another perspective to really see what is limiting us. And if we still feel blocked, psychotherapy serves a similar purpose to expand our thoughts and feelings of empathy.

Working with patients like Benjamin and Katrina, as well as my time in India, helped me wonder how some of the structural systems in our society were set up all wrong. Of course, now isn't the only time in history of the world with these inequities—we've seen these issues for many centuries. The good news is we have worked to right many of those historical wrongs. An example would be women not having the right to vote or own property until 1920 in the U.S., while women still don't have that right in many countries. If our *humanity* is what we all have in common, our structural systems should reflect that. I've never felt this more deeply than after the experience I had with Benjamin and Katrina.

One of the theses of this book is to highlight current unresolved structural problems, whether they are internalized psychological blocks, or external blocks within the system. What we eat exemplifies these blocks. I understand Western society has accepted eating processed meat and ultra-processed foods as part of our cultural norm. These choices have become habits and determined their availability, and we have reinforced this behavior for generations.

But now that we have the science on how unhealthy these *food products* are, are we ready to right the wrongs in what we label *foods* for humans? Hopefully, with this book, we can allow ourselves to honestly re-evaluate what we consider normal. Are packaged ultra-processed foods going to continue to be the norm, or are we going to challenge the status quo? Are we going to address the hold our culture has on our health and the health of the planet?

In order to delve into these questions more, let's first discuss how we change our individual behavior. I propose a comprehensive model encompassing concepts discussed thus far in this book. I call this the *Restack* Model of Change as discussed in the next chapter.

Part D: Solutions for Everyone

Chapter 9: *Restack* Model of Change

Right now, we often look at treatment in a siloed way. We say, "Do this for your heart health, do this for your kidney health, and do that for your liver health." But there are things we can do to support the health of all our body's systems. Our body's systems are all connected.

In lifestyle psychiatry, we've identified six overarching health factors, which we call the *six pillars of lifestyle psychiatry*: nutrition, restorative sleep, physical activity, stress management, connectedness, and minimizing toxic substances.[230] We'll discuss each of these in more detail later in the following chapters, but first let's consider a case highlighting behavioral change.

A Case of Lifestyle Factors in Depression and Anxiety

Abby, a 35-year-old female, had been diagnosed with depression when she was 21 years old. She was treated with medication, started feeling better, and then stopped the medication after a year. When she was 24, she became depressed again, this time with the added symptom of anxiety. She started taking medication again and her anxiety was better. From the ages of 29 to 34, she developed reflux, chronic constipation, and trouble sleeping, for which she was prescribed medication.

When I started working with Abby, we talked about how improving any specific lifestyle factor could potentially alter multiple problems she was experiencing. I mentioned the six pillars of lifestyle psychiatry to gauge which one she felt most comfortable addressing first. We talked about how adding physical movement to her day may help her depression. Additionally, we discussed how dietary changes could improve her gut microbiota, which may lessen her reflux and chronic constipation. I made it clear that it was her choice which, if any, of the pillars she would initially tackle.

Abby decided to work on decreasing consumption of ultra-processed food and adding 10 minutes of movement every morning for at least 60 minutes a week. She felt these goals were challenging and devoting 10 minutes to movement each day could be enjoyable. While the goal of decreasing ultra-processed foods in her diet was general, the exercise goals were specific. She identified a specific area in a room to exercise, as well as a support person whom she could touch base with regularly. Over 10 months, she slowly built on these lifestyle interventions, and many of her symptoms progressively improved. Abby started feeling better and thinking more clearly.

While Abby had a formal mental health diagnosis, this isn't necessary for a lifestyle psychiatry approach to be useful. The concept of mental health falls between a spectrum of diagnosed mental illness and undiagnosed mental suffering. Our ability to function in the world is called *functional impairment*. In order to make a formal diagnosis, psychiatrists look for impaired functioning and distress in addition to a threshold number of symptoms and their duration. In my case, I have never had a formal mental health diagnosis. But as is obvious, I have had numerous anxious and depressed feelings, which I've clearly discussed throughout this book. Indeed, I was still suffering.

Globally we spend billions of dollars on *treating* the symptoms of chronic diseases, both mental and physical. However, if we did better at *prevention* or treating those of us suffering without a formal diagnosis, it could ultimately cost less over time and lead to better health outcomes.[231]

Honoring Our Individual Lived Experiences and External Factors in Setting Goals

While there are many barriers and aspects to consider, including emotional, cognitive, and personality traits as described in previous chapters, ultimately, we have to be ready to effectuate an action in order to change behavior. Without recognizing the social determinants of health, trauma, etc., addressing behavior change often does not work, and leads to people being discouraged. This whole book examines the key components of behavior change, but the question is "What is the individual goal and how do we get from identifying the goal to changing our behavior?" The rest of this chapter will focus on these core components of goal setting. Which include: preparation, refining and setting your goal, identifying our "Why?," creating an action plan, using healthy coping strategies, bolstering confidence, and periodic check-ins with follow-ups.

The Importance of Fitting the Behavior Change Model with the Individual

Behavior change cannot be standardized to be a one-size-fits-all for every person. Let me repeat. Many of our failures in changing our behavior are related to this reductionist approach to behavior change strategies. As reiterated multiple times in this book, behavior change necessarily involves addressing our internalized and externalized barriers with grace and understanding. In addition, hundreds of different techniques to change behavior have been studied in the scientific literature. Of these, numerous different mechanisms of action have been postulated to be useful for individuals. It is hard to know from the research data, which one is the right one for a specific person, or you as an individual. If you have failed in changing your behavior, it may mean that the one you tried, the chosen technique, wasn't the right one for you. Even if it were the right technique, the data is clear -- it's not one technique in isolation that is needed. It's a sequential process layering many different techniques together to create your individual strategy for combating the behavior you want to change. And in fact, what works for you at one period of your life may not work during another. In Chapter 16: Beyond Self-Help we point out that not all therapists look at help in the same model, and therefore, if you don't do well with one therapist, it doesn't mean you are beyond help. It's just the behavioral change model being used didn't work for you at this time for this situation.

A Note on the Limitations of SMART Goals

The use of the acronym SMART goals has become so commonplace with many clinicians, especially in the sports and lifestyle medicine movements. But like with anything that becomes commonplace, such as "walking 10,000 steps a day" or "drinking 8 cups of water per day," just because it's commonplace doesn't mean it's accurate/factual scientific data. SMART goals were originally identified in 1981 as an acronym in an article published by a business consultant, George Doran.[232] He described SMART (Specific, Measurable, Assignable, Realistic, and Time Related) as an easy way to remember management goals and objectives in the business world.

What is the data to support SMART being scientifically valid? How did SMART goals become used by the American College of Sports Medicine, the NHS Health Trainer Book, and multiple other organizations, as the appropriate acronym for setting goals for behavior change? I must confess that, until recently, I hadn't questioned the validity of using the SMART acronym to develop goals for patients, because its use was so ubiquitous. After reviewing the scientific evidence, it is now my belief that blanketly using SMART goals for all individuals in all goal-setting situations is ill-advised for the following reasons:[232]

1. The use of SMART goals is not based on scientific data.
2. There is overlap within the SMART criteria.

3. For physical activity, the data supports that goals should be challenging.
4. SMART goals are not being used towards the original intention.
5. There are potential harmful effects for individuals who are overall inactive.

For example, in one study, SMART goals were noted to be detrimental for physical activity goals. The study suggests that the emotional response during activity is indicative of whether the person will exercise again.[233] Based on this information, what is the right approach for you? This is going to require a little bit of investigation and thought on your part. If there were a magic formula, I promise I would spell it out clearly here. But there isn't. What we do know is psychologists are working to try to distill this down and multiple theories have emerged regarding behavioral change methods.

What Are the Theories About Behavior Change?

While it would be convenient for a simple answer on how to rewire our behavior, the thousands of theories that have been written about it point to a complex matrix of possibilities. Some of the most prominent theories for behavior change include the Social Cognitive Theory,[234] Stages of Change Theory,[235] Theory of Reasoned Action/Planned Behavior,[236] Self-Efficacy Theory,[237] Cognitive Dissonance Theory,[238] Self-Determination Theory,[239] etc. There are fundamental similarities and differences in these theories and how change happens for an individual. These theories have been developed from the mid-1900s to the 2010s, and include authors such as Bandura, Prochaska, Villcer, Ajzen, Fishbein, and Rogers.

Describing each of these theories is beyond the scope of this book, but curious minds are encouraged to read the cited papers for further information.

Making Behavioral Changes

Many of us struggle with making changes in our lives, haunted by an ever-present question: "How do we change our behavior?" By understanding and utilizing the chapters and concepts in this book, it will become clear that we have to take our personality traits, emotions, cognition, social determinants of health, and trauma into consideration in order to change our behavior. I would love for it to be as simple as "Just do it," but often, that is not the case. By incorporating all these aforementioned aspects, we are delving into the *human* aspect of behavior change. Before taking the first step, targeting a specific behavior we want to change, we need to individualize the approach to our human characteristics.

Research data shows it may be helpful to identify why we want to change. "Why?" can have multiple facets. One type of behavior change theory involves focusing on *intention*. After identifying our why, we need to then go deeper and understand our intention to act. For example, my "Why?" to exercise may be to reduce the effects of aging and bone loss by doing weight-bearing exercises. But, if we don't intend on doing it, then no matter how inspired our "Why?" is, reaching our goal will fail. Intention involves three major factors, according to behavior change theories. These three factors—attitude, social norms, and behavioral control—look at the likelihood of us performing the desired behavior, that is, our intention to perform.[240]

Factors In Behavioral Change

Attitude is a well-researched psychological term referring to our belief about our behavior. For example, if you want your loved one, Colleen, to stop smoking, your attitude does not matter, but Colleen's attitude does. She may want to continue to smoke, and therefore, sustained behavior change usually cannot happen. In theory, the person's attitude must reflect an intention to change the specific behavior. The behavior needs to be specific, and the belief in that specific behavior needs to be understood.

Social norms is an aspect where Colleen may take into consideration what other people believe about the smoking behavior. On one hand, you may want her to quit, but on the other hand, all her friends may smoke, so she may be displaying a conflicted intention to stop smoking.

The third component is *behavioral control*. This focuses on the person's belief about their ability to do a behavior. So in this example, Colleen needs to believe she can stop smoking in order for this aspect of intention to be present.

So of course, as mentioned earlier, these three parts of behavior change—attitude, social norms, and behavioral control—must incorporate the social determinants of health,[241] external and internal blocks which include aspects of our personality traits, emotions, and individual skills and thoughts. These will be factored into the comprehensive *Restack Model of Change* I will introduce later in this chapter.

Importance of Cognitive Dissonance in Behavioral Change

Also important in our thinking would be addressing the *cognitive dissonance* within ourselves[242]. Cognitive dissonance refers to the act of holding two contradictory thoughts simultaneously and the internal conflicts that it creates. If we are presented with an idea, like "you are unhealthy if you smoke cigarettes," and our internal self-concept is that "I smoke cigarettes because the most loving person I knew, my uncle Bernie, smoked cigarettes," then cognitive dissonance may be created when someone asks you to stop smoking, due to its adverse health effects because it's unhealthy. The belief may be true or not true. This is not about arguing what is right or wrong, but understanding that making behavior change will be very difficult unless dissonance is resolved or softened in some way.

Willingness to Change

Some of us approach change head-on and are energized by it, which we call early adopters. Others of us are late to the game or struggle in our willingness to change. There's a spectrum in between those two. These are core parts of who we are and need to be taken into account as we're thinking about changing our behavior.

Belief in Ourselves

Another major factor that we would need to reflect on is if we are someone who is good at organizing ourselves and are skilled in following through a course of action to get the outcome we want. This basically is, "do we view ourselves as someone with *self-efficacy*?"[243] This concept refers to our internal confidence and belief that we can accomplish or attain certain things in our lives, and is intrinsically connected with our ability to achieve the goals that we set for ourselves. Often, our ability to motivate ourselves with the needed emotional state depends upon how we view ourselves as someone who can change. That is, our belief in our ability to produce an action matters the most.

Health Belief Model

Why, knowing what we know, don't we take more action for our health?

Many of us have known from childhood how important a healthy lifestyle is, but still struggle to implement the practices. The Health Belief Model is a theory to better understand why, even with the knowledge of how important healthy lifestyle practices are, we may not follow through. In this chapter, we will delve into factors we need to modify, and how those changes can be implemented to successfully change our behavior with a *Restack*. In my *Restack Model of Change*, I incorporated the transtheoretical model of change, the Health Belief Model, and other concepts from this book on *Restack* to operationalize healthy behaviors.

Components of the Health Belief Model

The Health Belief Model's central tenet stresses the factors directly affecting our likelihood to engage in healthy behaviors. Maximum engagement occurs when the threat of getting a disease and our trust in the recommendations for prevention are urgent enough.[244,245] This concept is not about increasing our knowledge, but about breaking the cycle of not sustaining change.

The model comprises six components which are listed in Rx 9.1 in the first column. Answer the questions in the second column to identify and consider these components for yourself.

Often, people are told the reason they don't engage in healthy behaviors is because they're simply not motivated. I disagree with this approach since motivation isn't the catch-all problem for all people. The Health Belief Model helps us identify aspects of our beliefs so that we can address the barriers that may be present.

Our Behavior Also Impacts Society

As we consider the many important aspects of behavior change, it's important to also consider how our behavior can impact society as well. Do we, for example, feel a personal obligation to the environment and, therefore, want to help make local parks safer for the community?

Or, do we want to do better with recycling plastics? Is societal pressure not significant enough for us to change this behavior, so we continue to throw everything into the trash that's going to the landfills? Many individuals could feel moved or inspired by social issues whereas these same issues could serve as barriers for others–both reasons could either limit or jumpstart behavioral change.

℞ 9.1 What Are Your Beliefs About Your Health?
Prescription

Aspect of the Health Belief Model	Questions to Ask Yourself
Perceived concerns	Do you have any diseases that run in your family?
	Have you been told by your doctor that you have any health risks, such as diabetes, obesity, etc.?
	Are you concerned about any illness or potential illness for yourself?
Perceived severity	How severe are these issues for you and within your family?
Perceived benefits	Do you see any potential benefits from engaging in healthy lifestyle habits?
Perceived mental blocks and external barriers	What are the mental blocks or external barriers keeping you from adopting healthier habits?
	Review Chapters 3-8 and brainstorm some ways to overcome the blocks.
Helpful guidance	Do you have access to resources that may help you make changes?
	Are there friends or family members whom you could talk to about their experiences with a similar health issue?
Taking action	Do you believe you can change your habits or lifestyle?
	List the action you hope to take and how you will incorporate it into your routine.

For me, I reflect back to the times when I was emotionally overwhelmed with my life and so busy that adding one more thing to my plate seemed overwhelming. During those periods, I'm not proud to say that I used single-use plastics and did not recycle. Cognitively, I knew the

182

importance in the 1980s of these behaviors and its impact on society, but I wasn't in a position to live true to my knowledge. So now, as an advocate and a strong believer in the importance of planetary health, how do I reconcile my younger self to my current self? Being true to who I am and being honest about my limitations is the only path forward that works for me. I was doing the best that I could, and now, I am grounded with the knowledge that I am able to do more. I can be true in my actions to my beliefs and not just "talk the talk," but also "walk the walk."

Transtheoretical Model of Change

Overall, as we're thinking about a specific behavior we want to change, we need to understand our intention and address our cognitive dissonance, willingness to change, and our assurance in ourselves being able to make the change—these all lead us to developing an intention and beliefs which must be addressed in addition to our "why." This has been described by Prochaska as the Transtheoretical Model of Change, involving progressing from the six stages of change: precontemplation, contemplation, preparation, action, maintenance, and relapse.[255] These stages reflect the cognitive aspects of change that are important and are a piece of the puzzle of behavioral change, as seen in Figure 9.1.

Implementing Behavioral Change

How do we then move to implementing or changing our behavior?[246] There are several contributing factors that should be taken into account when setting goals for behavioral change. An initial factor could include focusing on what your individual needs are when setting a goal. Is it that you need more knowledge, commitment, ability, or resources to come to a decision? Then, the goal should involve these issues and include an achievable manner of incorporating them. For example, if you don't physically have the capacity to run 2 miles, then focusing on a goal specifically aimed at improving your physical abilities would be important. If your need for goal-setting is that you struggle with self-regulation or determination, then those need to be the criteria that are used.

Your goals can be specific or non-specific, depending upon what works for you. Additionally, goals should be challenging. Even if you don't achieve that challenge, setting a goal that is difficult to achieve tends to drive us further than settling on a more realistic or achievable goal. A more difficult task to achieve inspires additional involvement and ultimately, further motivation to conquer said objective, leading to enhanced desire to achieve behavioral change.

The Human Behavior Change Project

The Human Behavior Change Project (HBCP) is a collaboration between scientists that started in 2017.[247] They identified thousands of behavior change interventions and noted that over 100 papers on behavior change are published every week. The collaborative did sophisticated research modeling to develop a catalog of behavior change interventions. Some of the studies noted poor scientific rigor and others noted significant data on what technique would help with a specific change an individual is targeting.

If you do visit this website, please beware, there's a massive amount of information. I'm not suggesting that every reader of this book visit their website, but I'm highlighting this research so that you don't become discouraged if one intervention doesn't work for you. Changing behavior is complicated, but it's not beyond hope.

And while behavior change through self-help or therapy techniques may be the mainstay of the way we address our behavior change, there are many researchers looking at how behavior change can also occur directly on the brain via a molecular level, promoting neuroplastic growth. Current research explores how antidepressants, psilocybin, and other molecular compounds interact and change the brain at a cellular neuronal level.

Typically, clinicians will adopt their preferred behavior change techniques. How can someone know which one is useful for them? If you have not been successful in the past, maybe the wrong approach was part of the problem. In this chapter, I will highlight a few of them. If you are not successful in changing your behavior, please try a different approach. As stated earlier, the current research stresses that the approach needs to be individualized for each person.

Based on this data, my new model titled the *Restack Model of Change* takes into account the pillars of lifestyle medicine and who we are as individuals.

Setting a Goal — Preparation

Preparing to set a goal can involve a plethora of interpersonal factors. *Social/self-support* is an integral part of the goal-setting process—such as including friends/family already involved in our daily routines as accountability partners. For those of us with limited social connection, self-support via journal writing or other self-motivational means can be equally effective in keeping ourselves accountable. Ensuring the goal is *important* to us is a pivotal step in goal-setting, as is enlisting the people around us to understand the importance of these goals and why we hope to change our behavior.[248]

Another key part of preparation is *identifying your goals*, or understanding specifically what you hope to achieve and how that looks for you specifically.[249] For example, if you don't have the physical ability to run 2 miles, then focusing on a goal specifically addressing your ability would be important. At the beginning of setting a goal, being too specific may interfere with achieving your goal. Flexibility is the key to this step.[250] If your reason for setting goals is that you struggle with self-regulation or determination, then those need to be the criteria that are used. The final step of preparation is to *reflect*—why haven't previous attempts to change behavior worked? What techniques have been effective for you? What are things that haven't stuck long-term? Reflecting on prior experience and understanding what does and does not work for you is critical in maintaining long-term behavior change.

Components of Goal Setting

There are a number of nuances to goal-setting we must consider. One crucial element is choosing *challenging goals* to work toward.[251] This may seem counterintuitive at first glance but in actuality, even if you don't achieve the challenging goal, setting a goal that is difficult to achieve tends to drive us further than just settling on a more realistic or achievable goal. A more difficult task to achieve inspires additional involvement and ultimately, further motivation to conquer said objective, leading to enhanced desire to achieve behavioral change.

Hopefully, you are also choosing *enjoyable goals*, ones that will bring you incremental amounts of satisfaction, despite their relative level of difficulty. The goals can be either *specific or general*, depending on which approach works best for you. As we saw in Abby's case, decreasing ultra-processed foods in her diet was a more general goal while her exercise goal was very specific. And finally, consider setting *daily and weekly goals*, tasks you track each day and a broader overarching goal to work toward over the week.

Overall, considering these components of goal-setting will help you create more achievable goals for yourself, ensuring they do not fall by the wayside like the vague New Year's resolutions we often make for ourselves. Instead we can better prepare ourselves for long-term behavior change.

What is Your "Why?" for Change

Even if we remove many of the blocks mentioned earlier in the book, that doesn't automatically translate to change. Change is intricate and involves many factors, including knowing our "why."

Motivational interviewing (MI) is a technique used by many clinicians to help patients implement lifestyle interventions.[252] But it can also be applied as part of self-help or with the help of a coach. In MI, a therapist, physician, or coach helps the patient identify "why" they're making a lifestyle change, by engaging them in change talk about their "why" versus having the patient remain in sustain talk, which centers on the "why nots." Sustain talk means sticking with the status quo. Usually the "why" is emotional or has significant meaning. They will encourage the patient to think about the positive, then the negative consequences of the intended behavior change. Clinicians then ask the patient how this behavior change fits into their life goals. Finally, they will ask the patient if they *want* to make the change and how *confident* they are that they can make the change, on a scale from 1 to 10.[253]

Some examples of "why" include:
1. I want to get out of debt so I can buy a house one day.
2. I want to walk/run in a 5K race next year with my sister.
3. My partner has asthma. I want to stop smoking.
4. I want to live to see my grandchild grow up.
5. My parents died at an early age. I want to live longer.

Using Rx 9.2, you can use MI to develop readiness by establishing your "why" and working outward from that source of motivation.

R℞ 9.2 Developing Your "Why?"
Prescription

1. Identify a change you would like to make in your lifestyle.
2. Ask yourself, "Why?" Why do you want to make this change? Repeatedly drill down your why until you get to the depth and heart of the matter.
3. As identified in Rx 9.3, note your cognitive readiness for change.
4. If you are in the precontemplation or contemplation stages, do not begin your identified goal. You will likely not be successful. Refine your goal.
5. Use Rx 9.4 to set your goal.
6. Revisit and adjust your goal after a set timeframe.

The Science of Motivational Interviewing

Motivational interviewing (MI) serves many purposes to help us in our healing.[254] When a therapist creates an empathic environment during the sessions, this allows us to feel comfortable enough to self-reflect. The therapist should avoid being judgmental and interpreting our behaviors in a negative light.

MI is often used in tandem with the transtheoretical model of change. Both techniques are supported by research and have been adopted internationally for most types of psychotherapy and coaching. The techniques have also been used to treat multiple disorders, including addiction, diabetes, and cancer.

Are You Ready for Change? The *Restack Model of Change*

MI focuses on *developing* our readiness to change, while the transtheoretical model focuses on *identifying* our readiness for change.

That readiness is gauged in multiple stages: precontemplation (not ready for change), contemplation (thinking about change), preparation (ready to change), action (doing the healthy behavior), and maintenance (staying on track with the healthy behavior).[255] Rx 9.3 contains questions you can ask yourself to evaluate your readiness to make changes.

R⊄ 9.3 Questions to Assess Your Cognitive Readiness for Change[255]
Prescription

Stage of Cognitive Change	Typical Statement Representing the Stage	Questions to Ask Yourself
Precontemplation	"I don't have a problem."	Am I aware of any behavior that is problematic or producing unhealthy consequences? Do I want to change the unhealthy behavior?
Contemplation	"I'm thinking about it."	Do I intend to take action to change the unhealthy behavior? Do I have a plan? Do I think the pros of changing the behavior outweigh the cons?
Preparation	"I'm ready to make a change."	Have I taken small steps toward changing the behavior? Do I believe that changing my behavior can lead to an overall healthier life?

While the popularly used concepts of motivational interviewing[254] and stages of change developed by Prochaska[255] are helpful, they don't include the very important mental blocks and external barriers we discussed in Chapters 3-8.

Creating an Action Plan

Organizing our goal-setting through an *action plan* is one way to improve the efficacy of our self-management to achieve behavioral change.[256] Through this plan we can identify strategies that will facilitate the most positive outcome from our goals. For instance, if your goal is to get more sleep, then an *action plan* would detail the various strategies such as scheduling relaxation time after work and limiting cell-phone use immediately before bedtime.

Another important element of the action plan is *modifying routine* in order to better achieve your goal. To go back to a prior example of running the 5K, if you hope to incorporate more cardio into your routine, ensuring you can make it to the gym before or after work in order to hit the treadmill is necessary to achieving this goal. However, if going to the gym is not part of an established routine, it may be difficult to incorporate into a packed schedule. One approach is habit stacking, where a person tries to link changed behaviors with something that the individual is already doing. It is also key to modify an existing routine in order to allow the time and flexibility to achieve your goals.[256]

Coping and Bolstering Confidence

The road to achieving our goal may include encountering some potholes and other obstacles on the road. Identifying environmental *barriers or blocks* and how to address them is another strategy for setting achievable goals. Some of these barriers include: time constraints, lack of support, and financial constraints (many of these factors are discussed in Chapters 7 and 8).

A major factor to reflect on is whether we are adept at organizing ourselves and capable of following through on actions to achieve our desired outcomes. Essentially, the question boils down to "Do we view ourselves as someone with *self-efficacy*?" This concept refers to our internal confidence and belief that we can accomplish or attain certain things in our lives, and is intrinsically connected with our ability to achieve goals we set ourselves.[257] Often, our ability to motivate ourselves with the needed emotional state depends upon how we view ourselves as someone who can change. That is, our belief in our ability to produce an action matters the most.

Assessing if *confidence* is meaningfully affecting your behavior change goal is critical. Are you confident in your ability to achieve your goal? And if the answer is no, why not? The following strategies can aid in improving confidence and removing barriers from your goals:

- Seeking solutions to situations or problems
- *Seeking resources that may help you achieve your goal* (a variety of helpful resources are available at giamerlo.com)
- *Using healthy coping strategies*: When facing difficult situations, healthy coping strategies help maintain calm (this is discussed further in Chapter 13, Rx 13.2, & Table 4.2)

Employing healthy coping strategies is helpful for many in the midst of behavior change. These strategies, summarized in Table 4.2, include *positive cognitive restructuring, problem solving, seeking support*, and *distraction. Positive cognitive restructuring* refers to active attempts to change one's view of a stressful situation, utilizing positive thinking or working to minimize distress in order to see a different side of the situation.[258] *Problem solving* highlights strategies used to address underlying stressors, including planning, logical analysis, and determination.

Seeking support is integral to behavior change, looking within our social circles, colleagues, or spiritual organizations for positive feedback, advice, and comfort. *Distraction* also proves a useful tool when dealing with a stressful situation by shifting to a different, more pleasurable activity, like spending time with friends, exercising, reading for pleasure, or whatever we find enjoyable in our personal lives. Put together, these strategies function to maintain calm in the face of stressors activated over the course of goal-setting and behavior change.[259]

Additionally, it is both natural and necessary to practice self-compassion throughout the process and acknowledge that we may not be in the exact place we hoped for in terms of achieving our goals.[260] As can be seen over the course of this book, there are myriad ways to affect behavior change. We should allow ourselves grace when things do not go exactly as planned. Below, we will review a goal-setting example in order to get more comfortable with the process.

A Case of Setting a Goal

Sylvia was excited about her daughter, Rose's high school graduation, occurring in about a year's time. She had been saving a dress that belonged to her mother for this special occasion. She desperately wanted to wear it but realized that the dress was a few sizes too small for her. She mentioned her desire to Rose and to her sister, who were not only excited about this prospect of Sylvia wearing the dress but also understood the emotional importance that by wearing the dress to graduation, Rose's grandmother would be there in spirit. She recalled other occasions she tried to wear this dress since her mother's passing 15 years ago. She got close one time to fitting into it and remembered that exercising with her neighbor and cooking a few more meals at home every week were really helpful.

Sylvia identified a goal she thought was challenging, but within her ability to fast-walk in the neighborhood for 30 minutes a day. She realized that a more vigorous activity would not be attainable. She was looking forward to the prospect of walking, and enlisted her neighbor, who excitedly agreed to walk with her every morning. Sylvia also decided to go shopping twice a week on her way home from work, so that she could buy her favorite seasonal vegetables to increase the number of times she cooks per week.

She began to notice a change in her body and with it getting healthier, she came to my office and said, "I'm having so much fun! Maybe we need to change the goal because getting into my dress is just not as important as before." She had a vibrancy and glow about her. Sylvia realized, as she was planning for this new venture, that fitting into the dress was a good reason to start, but really she also wanted to do it for herself because she's been feeling less energetic and more sluggish most days. Thereby, she revised and refined her "Why?" She reflected on the fond memories of the energy and improved mood she felt when she was eating better and engaging in daily physical activity in the past.

As she thought about her past attempts to have a better lifestyle, she remembered the discouragement she felt when her weight did not change on the scale for a few weeks. She decided she was not going to weigh herself–this time, it's about feeling better. Rose suggested they plan a weekly game night where they could discuss and celebrate Sylvia's successes. Sylvia made a plan to revisit her physical activity goal and her diet goal every month on the first of the month, so that she would be ready for Rose's graduation in 12 short months. She anticipates adding weight training, and some stretching sessions by month two to keep the goals difficult and challenging and to help maintain her motivation.

Periodic Check-Ins and Follow-Up

Check-ins and follow-ups are helpful tools to gauge progress and ensure we are listening to ourselves over the course of the process. One manner of checking-in with ourselves is *alignment*, or reviewing the goal and ensuring the parameters of the intervention are still consistent with the intended outcome. Another important step is to *evaluate confidence* in our ability to achieve the original goal we set. If confidence in ourselves is waning or if we feel disconnected from the goal, steps must be taken to either adjust the goal or bolster self-confidence.

Feedback from either our social support group or self-evaluation over the course of the process is another way to follow-up with our original goal-setting. Asking ourselves how we're doing, and if we are being challenged enough or being too challenged, are all questions that should be asked in order to find out whether the parameters for our goals should be altered in some way.[261]

Using Rx 9.4, set a goal for yourself.[257-262] What behavior do you want to address?

Sustaining Change

Once a goal is set, how do we then sustain change? Sustaining change involves revising your goals, taking action, maintaining your changed goals, getting back on track after a potential relapse, and *Restack*-ing as needed.

Oftentimes, your goals need to be revised after you set your goal and receive feedback. Other times, the goals may need to be revised because your needs changed or your goals are not challenging anymore. The action phase after revising the goals serves to help acquire new healthy habits and potentially use new coping strategies. Attending to our feelings during the action phase is especially important to consider. After a period of time, the maintenance phase is achieved. Maintenance involves changing our thoughts and emotions, addressing our barriers and blocks, and using healthy coping strategies.

R̶X̶ 9.4 Setting a Goal[257-262]
Prescription

1. **Preparation**
   a. **Social or self-support**: Enlist family and friend support for social support or use a journal to help with self-support.
   b. **Importance of activity**: Understand why you and others view the activity you're trying to change as important.
   c. **Identify your goal(s)**: Identify your goal(s) that you want to achieve.
   d. **Reflect**: Reflect on previous attempts to change the behavior. What were some techniques that worked, though they may not have stuck long-term?
2. **Your Goal**
   a. **Challenging goals**: Identify goals that are challenging and difficult, but do not exceed your capabilities.
   b. **Enjoyable goals**: Consider goals that are enjoyable and bring you pleasure.
   c. **General or specific goals**: The goal can be specific or general, depending upon what works better for you.
   d. **Daily and weekly goals**: Consider coming up with goals for each day, in addition to goals for each week.
   e. **Reviewing your "Why?"**: Consider goals that are important and personally meaningful.
3. **Action Plan**
   a. **Strategies**: Identify intervention strategies.
   b. **Modifying routine**: Identify ideas on how to change your routine in order to achieve your goal.
4. **Coping**
   a. **Healthy coping strategies**: Make a decision to employ more healthy vs. unhealthy coping strategies. Healthy coping resources are discussed further in Chapter 13, Rx 13.2, and Table 4.2.
   b. **Barriers**: Identify environmental barriers or blocks and how to address them, such as time constraints, lack of support, or financial constraints. These are discussed in Chapters 7 and 8.
   c. **Confidence**: Consider ways to bolster your confidence in achieving your goal and removing barriers:
      i. Seeking resources that may help you achieve your goal. Resources are available on my website giamerlo.com.
      ii. Be consistent in putting in the effort and sticking to your goals.
   d. **Self-compassion**: Acknowledge that feeling like you're not exactly where you want to be in this process is normal. Give yourself grace.
5. **Follow-Up**
   a. **Alignment**: Review the focus on the goal and make sure the intervention is aligned.
   b. **Evaluate-confidence:** Utilize confidence-boosting strategies, such as positive self-talk and social support.
   c. **Feedback**: Receive feedback from social support or review progress with self-evaluation on advancement in behavioral change.

If you get off track after a period of sustained change and fall into relapse, use the concepts in this book to assess your potential mental blocks and external barriers that may be interfering with maintaining your goal. Ask yourself if you've been triggered emotionally or if you have conflicting feelings or thoughts concerning your goals. As you reflect on the reasons for your relapse, you may need to go back to the beginning of the Restack Model of Change and readdress new emotions, thoughts, personality traits, and traumas that were triggered. Though it seems like a big task, rest assured that these revisiting of our blocks and barriers often gets easier and quicker with repetition and time. You may find that sometimes, you don't need to start from the beginning after a relapse and can get back on track by the process of increasing your awareness or resetting your goals. These options after relapse are graphically depicted in Figure 9.1.

In Rx 9.5, [257-262] review the stages of sustaining change. Typical statements representing the stage and questions that you can ask yourself are included to help you identify your current stage.

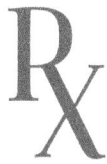

R⟨ 9.5 **Sustaining Change**[257-262]

Prescription

Stage of Sustaining Change	Typical Statement Representing the Stage	Questions to Ask Yourself
Revising Goals	"I'm updating my goals to meet my current needs."	Are my goals still challenging? Have I identified new goals that better align with my current needs? Have there been changes in my emotions and thoughts warranting goal revision?
Action	"I'm taking action."	Have I modified my unhealthy behavior for a short period of time? Have I acquired new healthy habits? Am I continuing to use healthy coping strategies and staying connected to my feelings?
Maintenance	"I'm doing it."	Has my unhealthy behavior changed? Have I sustained the change long-term? Do I intend to maintain the behavior change going forward?
Relapse	"I'm off track."	Have I fallen back into the unhealthy behavior? Has the temptation become too strong or overpowering? How can I get back on track?
Restack	"I'm assessing my mental blocks and external barriers that are interfering with maintaining my goal."	Have I been triggered emotionally, leading to changes in my coping strategies? Am I employing personality traits that may be interfering with my success? Do I have conflicted feelings and/or thoughts concerning my goal? Am I aware of emotions, thoughts, and behaviors leading to my relapse?

Putting It All Together: The *Restack Model of Change*

The revised model of change, titled *Restack Model of Change*, is summarized in Figure 9.1.[241-256] Please note, in this figure, the contents in Chapters 3-8 are depicted in the gray boxes. In most other models of change, the cognitive aspects of behavioral change are the ones that are of focus. Indeed, cognitive aspects of behavioral change are important. But as may be obvious from this book, I find that cognitive factors are one piece of the puzzle for lasting change. The other pieces include our emotion regulation, our internalized trauma, our environmental barriers, our work-related burnout, and our personality traits. Many patients have felt defeated if they don't succeed by focusing just on the cognitive. In this proposed model, using the Rx's presented in this book and addressing those blocks and barriers through a *Restack*, we then can move forward to addressing our conflicting feelings and thoughts, increasing our awareness, addressing our attitude, perceived norms, self-efficacy, and beliefs, as previously described. Then we are ready to set our goals with attention, take action, change our behavior, and move into the maintenance phase after a period of time. If and when we relapse, we can revisit our barriers and blocks and enter the *Restack Model of Change* at different points.

- Are your emotions, thoughts, and triggers activated and giving you trouble? If yes, go back to Chapters 3-6 and review the figures and Rx's until you develop some clarity and calmness. If no, proceed to the next step.
- Are you in need of increasing your awareness of your emotions, thoughts, and behaviors? If yes, use the Rx's in Chapters 3-6 that focus on increasing your awareness, especially Rx 3.1, Rx 4.1, Rx 5.1, and the Rx's on personality traits that you identified are relevant to you. If no, proceed to the next step.
- Do your goals need to be refined because of your relapse to be more consistent with your current needs? If yes, review Rx 9.2-9.4 and develop a new goal(s).

FIGURE 9.1 *RESTACK* MODEL OF CHANGE [241-256]

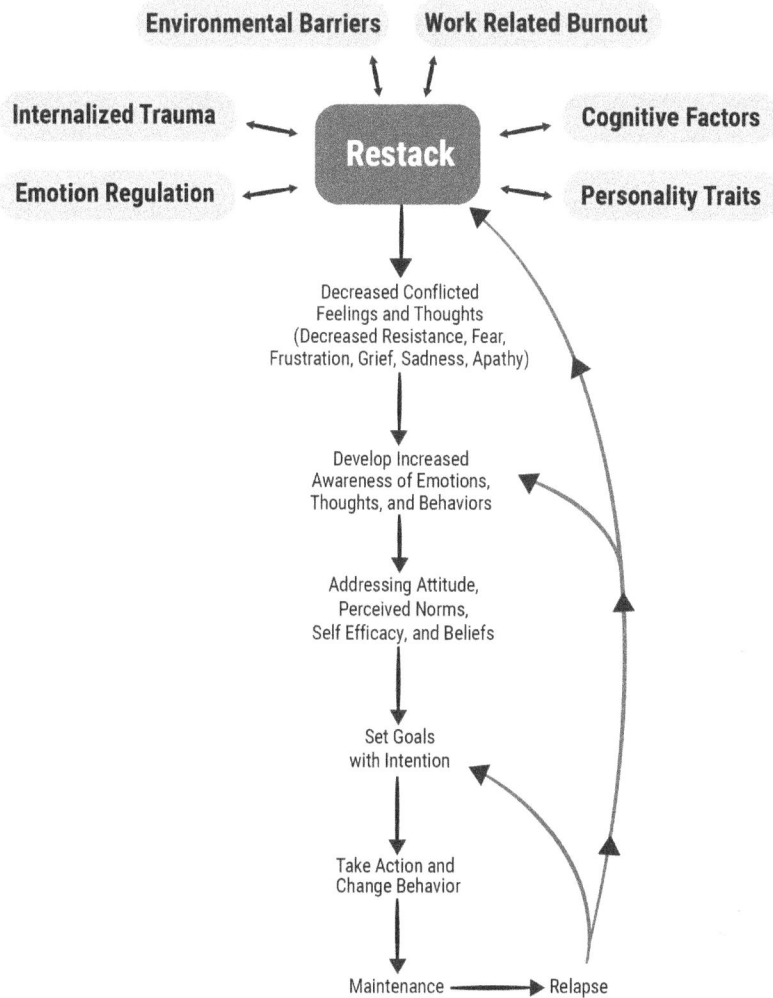

Environmental Barriers

Work Related Burnout

Internalized Trauma

Cognitive Factors

Emotion Regulation

Restack

Personality Traits

Decreased Conflicted
Feelings and Thoughts
(Decreased Resistance, Fear,
Frustration, Grief, Sadness, Apathy)

Develop Increased
Awareness of Emotions,
Thoughts, and Behaviors

Addressing Attitude,
Perceived Norms,
Self Efficacy, and Beliefs

Set Goals
with Intention

Take Action and
Change Behavior

Maintenance ⟶ Relapse

According to this Model, once we reach a sufficient level of readiness, then we should embark on a process of trying to change behavior. For example, attempting to quit smoking when someone is clearly in the precontemplation phase is doomed to fail oftentimes because it's not their personal goal but forced on them by others. The Model gives us many opportunities to show ourselves self-compassion, and address, if possible, these internal and external barriers. As we begin the process, it is important to show ourselves self-compassion. Each step of the process will present challenges where we may need to exit the cycle and address internal and external barriers before returning to the cycle.

A Case of the *Restack Model of Change* in Action

Irina is a 33-year-old chef who initially expressed that her husband wanted her to quit smoking before they tried to conceive. When she came to my office, she said, "I enjoy smoking, and it's my social outlet with friends." She was clearly in the precontemplation stage. Irina spoke of her fears of losing friends and her lifelong struggle with needing to fit in. She was able to relate this back to bullying that she experienced in middle school, which was around the time she originally started smoking. She recognized smoking as a coping strategy and feared, "I'm gonna be a hot mess if I stop." She suggested that she didn't know how to cope with stress without smoking. Her mental blocks–including trauma, emotion regulation, and her need for social connection–all needed to be addressed before she could move into the contemplation stage. While the transtheoretical model of change focuses on thoughts, the *Restack Model of Change* incorporates emotions, mental blocks, and external barriers.

Irina came in with external "motivations" to quit smoking, such as a desire to please her husband and wanting to have a healthy baby. Yet, at this point, she had not yet seriously considered change. Addressing her emotional blocks, her fears of losing control, and her traumas was necessary to move into the contemplation stage. Often this is achieved by providing psychotherapy. Through the use of motivational interviewing (MI), cognitively, I helped Irina recognize the negative consequences of smoking. As she began to express reasons for wanting to quit—in her *own* words and desires, not her husband's—she transitioned into the contemplation stage with her psychological history not creating barriers for her.

In the preparation stage, Irina said, "I'd like to quit, and if I joined the volleyball league, I'd have a different social outlet to replace smoking with friends." Upon inquiry, she noted that she felt grounded and was using her breathing exercises as well as daily meditations to quell her fear and anxiety around social isolation and her trauma. She furthered her thinking by considering how she could incorporate exercise into her daily routine to prepare for playing volleyball at a more athletic level. Ideas she came up with were going up and down the stairs multiple times a day as a break instead of scrolling the Internet. She identified people who could serve as emotional support for her in addition to the accountability partners of her sister and her daughter. For Irina, the people providing emotional support necessarily needed to be different. She felt uncomfortable sharing her psychological history with her daughter or sister, as she feared that it would cause more anxiety.

During the action stage, Irina spent 10 minutes a day going up and down the stairs and enjoyed journaling her feelings, thoughts, and progress. This usually brought her joy and took her mind away from smoking. Sometimes, she found herself being triggered by the physical activity and needed to review healthy coping strategies and stress-relieving ideas. Irina found that during the action stage, the coping strategies that she needed were different from the previous stages. She kept her mind open to explore different techniques like meditation and listening to music. After her sympathetic fear response got better with grounding techniques, she courageously was able to join the volleyball league without it causing her undue stress. With all the emotional and cognitive work that she did, she was ready to engage more readily with other members in the league. She reflected that, in the past, she would drop out of new social events for fear of being bullied. With her improved confidence, she began to have fun and saw herself as an "athlete."

In the maintenance stage, Irina continued her actions from the action stage, and utilized self-talk and affirmations to remind herself why she quit smoking. She continued to use grounding techniques, and her reliance on them was more self-directed without the fear she felt in the action stage.

Irina's continued abstinence (maintenance stage) from smoking also involved her getting support and reinforcement from her husband. She relapsed once and had a cigarette when she was at a work party. Upon reflection, she realized the smell of the smoke at the party was a trigger. In addition, when she mentioned this relapse at volleyball practice, someone said that they didn't know she stopped smoking because her clothes always smelled like smoke. Irina had no idea. Upon the advice of friends, she thoroughly cleaned all of her clothes with vinegar to remove the smell. She also decided to spend prep time preparing for work parties by creating an action plan of ideas to avoid smoking. After experimenting with a few different options, she found that chewing gum and using mints helped her stay away from cigarettes. This *Restack* allowed her to resume her maintenance.

Trauma-Sensitive Approach: Safety and Consent

For those of us dealing with trauma-related struggles, these frameworks need to be adapted. Instead of directly confronting our resistance when working through the transtheoretical model of change, it's better to "roll with" the resistance, support our self-efficacy, and strengthen the positive side of our double-edged sword.[263] For example we could focus on a skill that we want to acquire initially. The process of acquiring the skill will allow us to learn more about yourself, your feelings, and potential mental blocks. We need to be mindful of our need to feel safe, trust ourselves, and honor our truths. As discussed in Chapter 3 and Chapter 8, if we experience cultural and/or gender-related issues in our environment, engaging in self-talk and employing grace in the situation may be very therapeutic. Peer support and mutual self-help, whether through self-help groups or friends, can also offer significant benefits.

In my clinical practice, my trauma-sensitive approach to taking care of patients involved being mindful of language and being less direct. I remember an especially bright, astute, and articulate 45-year-old woman named Robin who, during her initial evaluation with me, appeared hesitant and shared her distrust of her previous psychiatrist. Toward the end of our session, I noted, "You mentioned earlier that you didn't have a good experience with your previous psychiatrist. That must be very difficult. I appreciate your trust in meeting with me today. Would you feel comfortable telling me what happened? That would help me avoid similar mistakes." The difference here is subtle yet important: I didn't ask Robin what happened; instead, I asked her if she would be comfortable telling me what happened. Essentially, I asked for Robin's consent. My aim is to establish safety and facilitate my patients' autonomy with this approach.

Is Our Diagnosis System "Healthy"?

In Chapter 2, we discussed the historical context of where we came from and where we are in the world of psychiatry in terms of different paradigms, methods of approach, and treatments. We expanded on this concept in this chapter and will continue to do so throughout the rest of the book.

The leading approach for psychiatric diagnosis is through the current volumes of *Diagnostic and Statistical Manual of Mental Disorders* and the *International Classification of Diseases*.[264] These two books approach psychiatry by categorizing symptoms into clusters and are very helpful in communicating symptoms amongst clinicians and patients alike. But, they are not solely based on science and not directly correlated to a region of the brain or underlying mechanisms. The books were compiled by a consensus panel of psychiatrists who negotiated on the meaning of the symptoms. While the scientific evidence was taken into consideration by the panel, often, there were differing interpretations of the data.

Does the way we conceptualize and categorize mental health diagnoses need to be revised? This is a question often debated among academic and clinical psychiatrists and psychologists. Because of this question, the field of transdiagnostic processes was developed by researchers.

What Is a Transdiagnostic Process?

Transdiagnostic processes offer a nascent, new, fresh, and burgeoning perspective. The term refers to a common mechanism present across various disorders, either as a factor predisposing to or perpetuating certain disease states.[265] It is a field offering a more inclusive and non-siloed approach to mental health and everyday health.

Is the current way of separating causes for disorders too simple and siloed? Many who do research in transdiagnostic processes think so. Additional research is potentially connecting overlapping mechanisms between many chronic diseases, such as the fatty liver preceding cirrhosis or the plaques in our arteries preceding heart disease.[266] If this connection is found to be true, then making changes to one risk factor can help in preventing a myriad of diseases.

It's important to remember that some risk factors can be changed, and some cannot. Genetic or anatomical risk factors, like an abnormality in the brain's blood vessels predisposing to an aneurysm, can't be changed with lifestyle. But quitting smoking, for example, can help prevent lung and heart diseases.

To be sure, the New Year's resolution you make every January could be the ticket to a *Restack*-ed you.

Conclusion

Prescriptions can be more than just pills.

In our healthcare system, we've found ourselves in a place where physicians only use prescriptions for medication. However, I'm proposing that physicians can also use prescriptions for positive health behaviors and activities. In this book, we've utilized these prescriptions (Rx's) for assessment, reflection, and actionable steps.

You can continue to use this book and the Rx's contained here to prescribe for yourself.

The question is often how to begin this process. To prescribe positive health behaviors, you need a way of assessing your degree of health in different areas of your lifestyle. We're going to discuss these lifestyle behaviors in six different buckets, which correspond to the six pillars of lifestyle psychiatry. We'll start with what we eat.

Chapter 10: Nutrition

I went against the doctor's advice and got better—for a while, anyway.

When I was in my early 30s, my bloodwork showed elevated lipids, including a cholesterol level of about 350, and the preventive cardiologist told me the only way to reduce it was with medication since only 10-15% of our cholesterol can be changed by diet.[267] I believed them, and the textbooks at the time also said the same. I tried about ten different medications with multiple side effects. These scary side effects included fasciculations (which are muscle twitches) and liver enzyme elevations. But then, I stopped taking the medication, stopped eating fast foods, and started exercising. I lost 30 pounds, and my cholesterol became normal. Yes, my cholesterol and all my lipid levels became normal. Without knowing it or meaning to, I stopped an inflammatory process. My doctors, who until this moment believed that only 10-15% of cholesterol could be changed by lifestyle interventions, were awestruck. As they were walking away from my exam room, I heard them excitedly talking about doing research based on my case.

At the same time I received the cholesterol diagnosis, I went to a rheumatologist because I had some vague joint pains. My labs showed high inflammatory markers pointing to Lupus.[268] I was devastated. After my initial cardiology appointment, I was imagining a life of heart attacks, strokes, and now this? Living with Lupus all my life? Fortunately, to everyone's amazement, all those markers went back to normal as well once I changed my diet and exercise habits and lost my extra weight.

Of course, the story is never that simple. This isn't a salvation narrative. I didn't stay healthy. On top of all the medical issues, I was also under an inordinate amount of stress. As a young physician with a child, I felt miserable and often worried excessively.

Eventually, I lost control of my lifestyle habits. I gained the weight back. And this *yo-yo* continued for decades, because the issue wasn't just lifestyle-related. The trauma and other blocks I wrote about in previous chapters held me back from fully engaging in a healthy lifestyle.

What's also important to understand is that my journey to health doesn't end with my cholesterol levels. As I've emphasized before, the relationship between mental and physical health is bidirectional. My stress, along with my anxious and depressed feelings, added to the complexity of my symptoms. Some data suggests decreasing cholesterol helps us think better, pointing to a connection between what happens in our brain and the state of our physical body.[269]

Plant-Based Diets Have Minimal to No Cholesterol

It's worth repeating as many times as we need to hear it: Whole food, plant-based foods have "several hundreds to thousands fold" less cholesterol than animal products.[270] Therefore, a good majority of our dietary cholesterol comes from animal-based foods.

Less than 1% of the population is genetically predisposed to high cholesterol, which can be diagnosed in at-risk family members via genetic testing.[271] Those individuals may not be able to get their cholesterol under control by any means except medication. But *most* of us can improve our cholesterol with diet. Even though I am genetically predisposed to high cholesterol, I could still use diet and exercise to reduce my cholesterol to normal numbers. If I can do it, those without a genetic predisposition can also do it.

For those of us with a genetic predisposition to high cholesterol, the liver produces excess cholesterol in our body. This by itself or with the added dietary cholesterol can lead to fatty liver. Even without a genetic predisposition to high cholesterol, having too many unhealthy fats in our diets can also lead to fatty liver. Of note, certain plant-based ultra-processed foods do interact within our body and elevate our cholesterol and/or other unhealthy fats, for example, trans fat.[272] The lesson here is, not all plant-based foods are the same. Though none of us are perfect, we should aim for as many whole food, plant-based foods as possible in our diet. Nonalcoholic fatty liver disease is one of the most common medical diagnoses, seen in about 25% of the population![273] It can often be treated and even reversed with diet and exercise if addressed early enough.[274]

In my case, my cholesterol and joint swelling can both be seen as related to inflammation. The inflammation is not only a risk factor for developing these conditions, but also part of the reason I continue to have high cholesterol and joint swelling–that is, the inflammation is an example of a transdiagnostic process.[275] While focusing on getting better by healthier eating, exercise, and losing weight is important, maybe we also need to work toward a better way to understand the causes and diagnosis of these seemingly disparate conditions.[276]

Hospital Food

The hospital where I worked as a resident had a McDonald's in the building, and for a long time that was my food of choice when I was on shift. It was cheap and readily available. In most hospitals in this country, after someone has, for example, knee replacement surgery, the only options available are high-fat ultra-processed foods, including sausage, hamburgers, and fried foods. There are over 6,000 hospitals in the United States, with over 34 million patients admitted to the hospital every year.[277] We need to do better for the clinicians and the patients in our healthcare system, to give them options supporting a lifestyle of healthy living.

The Healthcare System in the United States

The U.S. is both first and last in healthcare.

While we have the most expensive healthcare system in the world, when compared to the top six industrialized countries, the U.S. is last in terms of quality of life, health equity, and access to healthcare.[278] This dissonance is in large part because our healthcare system isn't designed, and doctors aren't trained, to implement lifestyle interventions such as healthy diet. These interventions would serve a preventative role, leading to lower healthcare costs and a better quality of life.

This problem spans beyond the healthcare system, though. The U.S. government subsidizes goods based on lobbying efforts, which means they subsidize products like ultra-processed foods and animal products from the dairy and meat industries.[279,280] Are these subsidized foods healthy? This chapter addresses the question of which foods (and food products) are healthy based on scientific evidence, *not* activism, politics, marketing, or sentiment.

Rx 10.1 Reflecting on Your Nutrition
Prescription

1. How many servings of fruit do you eat per day?
2. How many servings of vegetables do you eat per day?
3. Do you drink at least 8 cups of water per day?
4. How many 8-ounce cups of sugary drinks (such as soda, juice, or sports drinks) do you drink per day?
5. Do you add salt to most of your meals?
6. Do you eat processed meats (such as bacon, sausage, or hot dogs)? How many servings per day?
7. How many servings of packaged snacks do you consume per day?
8. Do you incorporate plant-based protein (such as nuts, legumes, beans, or tofu) into your diet?

In the last few decades in the U.S., only partially because of the whole food, plant-based movement, the consumption of dairy has decreased substantially, causing profits in affected industries to dwindle.[281] Large, multinational for-profit companies have been aggressive in using marketing terms like "plant-based," "vegan," and "health food," trying to capture a part of this new health market. But we need to read the labels, since many of these goods are still ultra-processed and have unhealthy additives. While consuming processed food products in moderation is okay, they are not the best options for the health of our bodies.

Before reading this chapter, reflect on your dietary patterns in Rx 10.1. This chapter will address the questions in the Rx, and your answers can point you in the direction of interventions to improve your nutrition and overall health.

As we begin the chapter, let's start the conversation with hydration. When considering nutrition, our thoughts usually go to macro and micro nutrients, proteins, fats, carbohydrates, and the like, but dehydration is one of the most common, poorly investigated, undertreated, nutritional problems.

Hydration, Underhydration, Dehydration, and Overhydration

Globally more than 50% of the world's population is not properly hydrated.[282]

The general recommendation to drink 8 glasses of water a day has been popularized and has become a part of common lore.[283] This guideline appears to have originated in 1945 with the U.S. Food and Nutrition Board with limited to no scientific data to support it.[284] Today, this attention to the need to drink adequate water daily has become so pervasive that we are desensitized to the message, often getting relegated to background noise. The unfortunate reality is that as a society, we are seriously underhydrated, with over 50% of the population worldwide not drinking enough water. Why is this important and what effects can we see as a result of an imbalance in our body's hydration?

The consequences of underhydration can be categorized as *acute* (lasting for just a few days) or *chronic* (long-term). *Acutely*, prolonged exercise, exposure to increased heat, and decreased water intake can lead to an immediate reduction of water in our body and cells. For example, with acute underhydration, just a few days can lead to a 48 oz loss of our body water content, which results in a 2% decrease in body weight.[285] In adults, it's estimated that this 2% decrease can lead to a 20% worsening in our physical performance and cognitive impairment in our immediate memory, attention to tasks, and mental acuity.[286] In children, even a 1-2% decrease in body weight fluids can result in significant impairment in cognitive functioning including confusion, irritability, and sluggishness. Athletes may lose, through sweat, between 6-10% of their water loss, resulting in increased heart rate to pump enough blood through our circulation.[287]

On the other hand, *chronic* underhydration may occur in otherwise healthy people who are not exposed to environmental conditions or vigorous exercise. This can occur through certain medications. Through chronic underhydration, they adapt to this state leading to cardiovascular effects including hypertension and kidney problems because the body tries to hold onto the water that it has. There is an increased risk of diabetes in the future, obesity, coronary artery disease, and faster aging. Interestingly, because of our body's adaptation to this chronic dehydration state, the labs that normally point to dehydration may be normal. Chronic dehydration can be difficult to detect and potentially dangerous long-term.[287]

A recent study suggested that over 90% of older patients over the age of 60 were dehydrated after fasting overnight. This was concerning for the health of our elderly and their risk for death by any cause (also known as all-cause mortality), which is correlated with the elevated plasma sodium levels as seen in dehydration.[288] In addition, heart failure, diabetes mellitus, obesity, coronary artery disease, and kidney function all are markers of hydration status.[287]

Diet can play a role in how much water we need to consume outside of solid foods. Ultimately our need for water is very individualized, depending on multiple factors, including composition of our diet, our physical activity, and sweating. A little-studied cause of underhydration is the role of ultra-processed foods in our diet. Ultra-processed foods are known to contain significantly less water and more salts than their whole food counterparts, and some researchers have suggested that historically over 70% of our water intake globally was from the water in our food.[289,290] With the shift of the increased amounts of ultra-processed foods in our diet, this balance may no longer hold as the recent literature suggests that about 20% of our fluid intake needs are coming from our solid foods.[290]

Whether we're underhydrated because of decreased consumption of water, increased consumption of ultra-processed foods, or other causes, the implications for our health acutely or chronically are strong. Other causes can include diseases that predispose to dehydration including diabetes, kidney disease, and taking medications like certain diuretics.[287]

No amount of change in our diet with nutrition is going to be effective in improving our health if we don't attend to the important task of adequate hydration.

As just mentioned, underhydration can be a serious health problem for individuals, but the opposite, *overhydration*, is rarely researched by scientists. Overhydration can occur from medical conditions that cause your body to retain water like liver disease, kidney problems, uncontrolled diabetes, congestive heart failure, and certain medications like diuretics. Polydipsia refers to the abnormal urge to drink fluid at all times. There are multiple causes of consuming too many fluids including compulsive water drinking, occurring in certain mental health conditions like anxiety, depression, and schizophrenia, leading to what is known as *psychogenic polydipsia*.[291,292] This appears to be mediated in the mesolimbic dopaminergic rewards system of the brain. Another type of polydipsia is called *social polydipsia* where people drink too much water for the health benefits. Social polydipsia can lead to bladder and kidney problems and in extreme cases, swelling of the brain. Chronic overhydration can also lead to an adaptive response of dry lips, decreased taste, polyuria, and kidney infections.[291] Because of these severe consequences of overhydration, multiple government authorities have released new guidelines to recommend that total water intake include all fluids consumed plus the water present in foods.[293]

As is with underhydration, overhydration can be acute and chronic. When we drink fluids because we are thirsty, it's associated with the activation of pleasure centers in the brain and is involuntary. Drinking to *thirst satiation* is pleasurable and involuntary, but once our intake of fluid is adequate, further consumption of fluids leads to an unpleasant feeling. This pleasure-displeasure balance is mediated in the brain in regions that are associated with swallowing, and the motor cortex of the brain.[289] A concept called *coached hydration* occurs when our normal bodies' signal for us to stop drinking is overwritten by a person being "coached" to drink more fluids.

Our hydration status affects our body in multiple ways and can affect us cognitively as well as physically. Though not usually considered a nutrition topic, another important aspect to consider is the concept of inflammation–the common pathway of many chronic diseases.

The Inflammatory Process in Our Bodies

Suboptimal diet is the #1 cause of mortality, according to the Global Burden of Disease.[294] But not only are people dying of food-related diseases—almost one-half of Americans are living with noncommunicable chronic disease, which severely impacts our quality of life. An estimated 7 of the 10 leading causes of death in the U.S. are chronic diseases.[295] The common pathway of these chronic diseases appears to be inflammation, which can be caused by the foods we eat.

Inflammation is our body trying to rid itself of foreign substances. When inflammatory cells become overburdened or overwhelmed, it can cause oxidative stress and collateral damage to tissues and organs.

What are these foreign substances? They include animal products like red and processed meat including hot dogs, bacon, lunch meats, and cured meats; refined grains like white bread, white rice, pasta, and breakfast cereals; as well as sweet snack foods, soda, sweetened drinks, and fried foods. These foods trigger inflammation in the body through a number of direct and indirect pathways. As a result, fat builds up in the arteries and leads to a chronic inflammatory state. This results in atherosclerosis, a thickening or hardening of the arteries because of plaque buildup, which puts us at risk for a heart attack.

A concerning new finding we're seeing in *young children* is fatty streaks in their blood vessels, the first stage of atherosclerosis and heart disease.[296] This is likely due to the increased intake of fatty foods and the increasing incidence of children suffering from excess weight and obesity.

Is our trajectory toward increasing rates of heart disease and chronic physical issues a *fait accompli*, or can we do something about it?

Preventing versus Reversing the Inflammatory Process

We can help *prevent* the inflammatory process by avoiding unhealthy foods. Conversely, if you already have the inflammatory process happening in your body—or like me, are not perfect in your food choices—you may be able to *reverse* this process by activating anti-inflammatory cytokines, which are produced by omega-3 fatty acids.[297] This is why foods rich in omega-3, like flax seed, walnuts, and brussels sprouts, are often recommended as sources of healthy fats.

What I just described are the direct pathways for inflammation in our body. More indirectly, inflammation is brought on by eating high-sugar foods that elevate blood sugar levels—this may eventually lead to insulin resistance and type 2 diabetes.[298] A high-calorie diet composed mostly of ultra-processed foods causes fat cells to secrete many hormones and substances that put our bodies in an inflammatory state. Inflammation, as we've discussed before, is the body's normal response to cuts, infections, or foreign substances entering the body. This means our bodies have numerous ways of expressing the inflammatory state. We may experience this as chronically feeling tired, swelling in our joints and joint pain like with arthritis, coughing and wheezing, feeling depressed or anxious, or a myriad of other symptoms.

When we understand our diet's influence on these inflammatory states, we can become empowered to act. In addition, eating whole foods helps us increase the phytonutrients in our diets. These phytonutrients are compounds with antioxidant and anti-inflammatory effects, shown to reduce risk of cancer, heart disease, and neurodegenerative diseases.[299]

The impact of removing inflammatory foods, while increasing phytonutrients, can be dramatic. Saray Stancic, a physician, in her book *What's Missing from Medicine,* writes about the eight years during which she experienced symptoms of multiple sclerosis, including pain, inflammation, and the inability to move.[300] Ultimately, she was able to completely reverse these symptoms with a whole food, plant-based diet. She went off all her medications and was able to run a marathon!

The SAD Diet: The Standard American Diet

How are we doing with eating anti-inflammatory foods? Research shows that Asia has the highest vegetable consumption, whereas research shows that less than 3% of Americans follow the guidelines of eating enough fruit and vegetables.[301] Most Americans follow a diet high in fats and sugar and low in fiber—a diet that's earned the unfortunate name SAD, which stands for the standard American diet. In the SAD diet, more than half the calories come from baked sweets, soft drinks, chips, candy, cheese, beef, and alcoholic beverages, which are all inflammatory.[302,303] While the SAD diet refers to the standard diet in America, a similar trend in diet is also seen globally, in about 30-50% of other countries.[304]

Ultra-Processed Foods

Ultra-processed foods are one of the biggest downfalls of our food system.

Between 50 and 60% of the foods Americans eat are ultra-processed foods, which are not actually foods but *food products*.[305] They're what we get when we process a food until almost all the nutrients are gone. Commercial canning in metal was practiced in the U.S. as early as 1812, but innovations in methods made it more commercially available after World War II.[306] This led to the mass production of convenience foods, like TV dinners and boxed cereals. These foods were exciting since they had a longer shelf life and were so easy to cook. This trajectory continued through the 1970s and '80s with the emergence of the fast-food industry and "supersized" portions, leading to increased caloric intakes, higher rates of obesity, and chronic diet-related diseases. Having shelf-stable products was seen as a huge added benefit historically. This led to economic efficiency since ultra-processed foods are cheaper for companies to produce, and they maximize company profits. Again, I would say these are not foods but are *food products*—something that mimics food but isn't really food. In addition, flavor enhancement makes these food products hyperpalatable, creating cravings and encouraging overconsumption.

What happens to food when it becomes processed? Four major types of food products are available for us to buy and consume, varying from whole foods (that are minimally processed) to ultra-processed foods as depicted in Figure 10.1: [307,308]

1. *Minimally processed or whole foods* retain their original nutritional content, and usually require cleaning during preparation and use minimal packaging. Minimally processed foods can be categorized into plant-based (fresh fruits, vegetables, nuts and seeds, beans, legumes, whole grains) and animal-based (fresh meats, fish, dairy products).
2. *Processed foods* have undergone preservation for convenience or to enhance taste. These include canned foods, frozen foods, dried fruits, and minimally processed meat (cut and packaged with trimming, marination, and/or seasoning).
3. Ultra-processed foods tend to be calorie-dense and nutrient-poor and have undergone significant processing with added sugars, fats, artificial flavors, and additives. These include snack foods, sugar beverages, fast foods, instant meals, and processed meats.
4. Culinary ingredients are usually included in the ultra-processed foods (bottle of ketchup or mustard), but some may be minimally processed (spices).

The Science of Ultra-Processed Foods

If you look at a food package and can't pronounce many of the ingredients, it is undoubtedly ultra-processed.

FIGURE 10.1 DIFFERENT TYPES OF FOOD PROCESSING [307, 308]

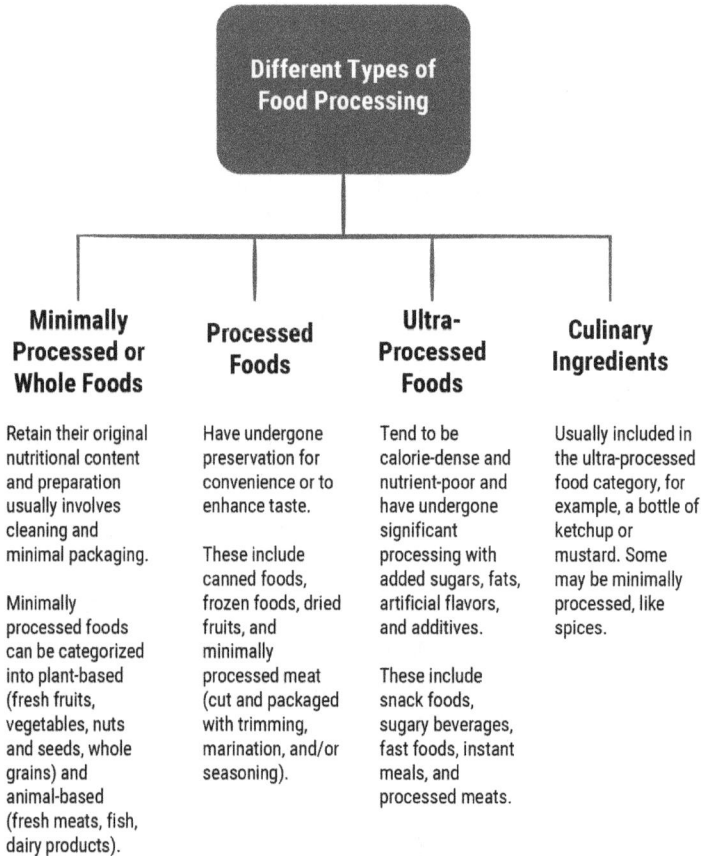

Different Types of Food Processing

Minimally Processed or Whole Foods

Retain their original nutritional content and preparation usually involves cleaning and minimal packaging.

Minimally processed foods can be categorized into plant-based (fresh fruits, vegetables, nuts and seeds, whole grains) and animal-based (fresh meats, fish, dairy products).

Processed Foods

Have undergone preservation for convenience or to enhance taste.

These include canned foods, frozen foods, dried fruits, and minimally processed meat (cut and packaged with trimming, marination, and/or seasoning).

Ultra-Processed Foods

Tend to be calorie-dense and nutrient-poor and have undergone significant processing with added sugars, fats, artificial flavors, and additives.

These include snack foods, sugary beverages, fast foods, instant meals, and processed meats.

Culinary Ingredients

Usually included in the ultra-processed food category, for example, a bottle of ketchup or mustard. Some may be minimally processed, like spices.

Ultra-processed foods have significant effects on the brain in multiple areas including cognition and mental health, mostly related to ingredients added during the processing (sugars, saturated fats, artificial additives).[309] The brain is responsible for appetite regulation, and this can be disrupted by two mechanisms: (1) Ultra-processed foods lack the dietary fiber that helps us feel full after a meal, and (2) Added sugars, salts, and saturated fats can also disrupt our appetite regulation mechanisms.[310] This is a result of the body's failure to release leptin, also known as the satiety hormone. These high amounts of sugars and saturated fats turn off our brain's ability to respond to leptin, a phenomenon called leptin resistance.[311]

Additionally, ultra-processed foods trigger dopamine release, which ultimately causes us to become desensitized to dopamine and need more to experience the same pleasure response over time.[312] The brain's reward pathways are stimulated by the added sugars, fats, and additives. We can develop cravings that lead to overeating and cognitive dysfunction, such as problems with memory, attention, and learning.[313]

As stated before, if we look at the back of a package and it has more than four or five ingredients, including words you can't pronounce, that's usually an ultra-processed food. This is the case even if the branding on the front says "vegan" or "plant-based." These words don't mean "healthy." So many of my patients report an *aha* moment when they start reading labels and understanding how many ultra-processed foods they've been eating without knowing. Let's not let the advertising fool us.

Food Is Medicine

An important saying is taking hold in medicine right now: "Food is medicine." Eating mostly whole and plant-based foods, while minimizing animal proteins and highly processed foods, is one of the best ways to avoid or combat inflammation. This conversation will continue in subsequent chapters on stress and exercise. Realistically, we're not going to be perfect, but if we eat more of these healthy foods, then we can "crowd out" unhealthy foods. "Crowding out" allows us to become fuller and feel satisfied with the healthy foods, and thus we eat less and less of the unhealthy and ultra-processed foods. When we discuss good nutrition, I'm focusing on risk reduction and trying to address the cause of poor health before the onset of disease. But even if someone has a disease, good nutrition can slow the progression of the disease, or sometimes even reverse it!

A Case of Mental Health and Ultra-Processed Foods: *Restack*-ing Our Blocks!

Nate was a 29-year-old male patient of mine who was finding it difficult to manage his symptoms of bipolar disorder. He was taking multiple medications he needed, which I strongly suggested he continue. We discussed his lifestyle along the six pillars of lifestyle psychiatry. Together, we were able to identify a few interventions that could help him stabilize on the medications he was prescribed. His diet consisted of over 80% ultra-processed foods. Just through education and helping him incorporate easy recipes with plant-based whole foods into his day-to-day, he began to think more clearly. I also encouraged limiting caffeine and alcohol and engaging in *mindful eating practices.* Mindful eating practices involve eating with intention and focusing on what we're eating while also minimizing distraction, tasting our food, and chewing our food until it's completely "mush." After a few months, he started feeling better on his medication. So, for him, the issue wasn't that the medications were wrong (he had tried multiple medications that didn't work over the years!), but his unhealthy lifestyle habits *blocked* the helpful effects of the medications.

Depression and Nutrition

Several studies have shown improved mood with dietary changes including the HELFIMED, SMILES, and AMMEND studies.[314-321] Based on these studies, the recommendations are to avoid ultra-processed foods and fast foods, while increasing intake of whole fruits and vegetables. Ultra-processed foods are associated with an increased risk of mental health symptoms, notably depression. Similarly, animal-based diets involve elevated amounts of L-carnitine, chlorine, and betaine, which once metabolized in the gut, are also linked to depression.[317]

So, What Does Good Nutrition Look Like?

The current U.S. Dietary Guidelines have four recommendations:[322]

- Consume nutrient-dense food. This means eating foods high in vitamins, minerals, and other health-promoting components with minimal added fats, sodium, and sugar.
- Eat within one's calorie needs with a balance of foods. Portion sizes should be restricted, and a variety of foods from all food groups should be consumed.
- Follow these recommendations across the entire lifespan, from childhood to old age. This is especially important since 40% of children in the U.S. right now meet the criteria for being overweight or obese.
- Limit foods with higher added sugar, sodium, and saturated fats, and limit alcohol intake.

While most people are aware of these basic nutritional factors, many of us have become so accustomed to hearing what we should do that sometimes we tune out the direct connection between the food we eat and its impact on our bodies.

When I was a young physician, I worked 14-hour days and had a young child. Preparing fresh food seemed like a huge burden. As I look back, I would say, at that time in my life, 90% of my diet was ultra-processed food. These foods are calorie-dense (see Figure 10.2), and I was in a cycle of eating mindlessly. The addictive properties of the high sugar, high salt foods made it difficult to control my consumption. I went from a "healthy" BMI of 22 to a hair under 30 in a few short years. In the medical field, a BMI of 30 and above is considered "obese," whereas a BMI from 25 to below 30 is considered "overweight." Once I was ready to take action, finding a way to break the cycle became my mantra. Over time, I found that cooking with my daughter and making it a fun activity wasn't a burden at all, but something we both looked forward to! Not only did cooking change my lifestyle, but it also helped me to refrain from eating ultra-processed foods such as microwavable meals or something from a fast food restaurant.

FIGURE 10.2 CALORIE DENSITY OF FOOD

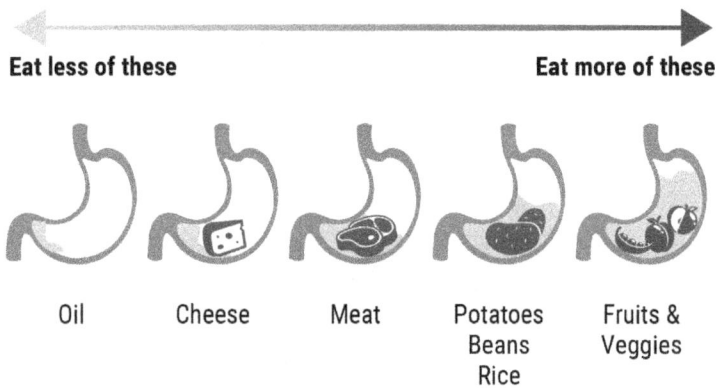

Eat less of these   **Eat more of these**

Oil   Cheese   Meat   Potatoes   Fruits &
                                            Beans   Veggies
                                            Rice

Please Note: If you eat more on the left, you will not feel full, so try to consume more on the right.

What Is Caloric Density of Food?

The *caloric density* of a food refers to the calorie content based on the food's weight or volume. Food with a high caloric density doesn't fill us as much because it takes up less space in our stomach. For example, two tablespoons of oil are about 240 calories. That would be the same as eating 3 cups of blueberries or 6 cups of broccoli or 40 cups of green leaf lettuce! In Figure 10.2, if you eat more foods on the left, such as the oils and cheese, you will not feel as full as you would if you consumed more of the fruits and vegetables on the right.

Fiber

Fiber is the silent hero of our health.

Still, 95% of Americans do not get enough fiber, which is necessary for the survival of our gut microbiota.[323] Fiber has been one of the most poorly understood nutrients since the beginning of nutrition research. When I went to medical school in the 1980s, most people thought fiber's only purpose was to help with regular bowel movements and was otherwise nonessential in our diets. Many of us still believe this. We were also taught fiber could cause nutrient depletion, meaning an inability to absorb certain foods.

Why is fiber so important? We have about 70 million organisms in our gut, called the gut microbiota. In the popular press and some academic papers, the words *microbiota* and *microbiome* are used interchangeably, though a microbiome is defined as the genetic material of all the microorganisms in the environment, and the microbiota is the living organism.[324] For the purposes of this book, I will be using the term microbiota.

Unhealthy microbiota in our gut are associated with diseases and thrive on ultra-processed foods and unhealthy foods. If we feed our gut microbiota fiber-rich foods, the healthy microbiota—called the probiota or *probiotics*—will propagate. So, the gut depends on fiber to maintain microbial diversity and promote the growth of healthy bacteria in our intestinal tract. By the way, this dietary fiber is also called *prebiotics*.

Fiber serves as energy for the beneficial bacteria we depend on for our bodies to work, both physically and mentally.

Why Do We Depend on Healthy Gut Organisms?

Many fiber sources are not digestible by humans because we lack the enzymes to digest them. Therefore, we are dependent on the bacteria in our gut to break down the fiber into short-chain fatty acids (SCFA) and butyrate, both of which are pivotal for reducing inflammation in our body.[325] The good news is many of the bacteria we house in our gut can be completely replaced in just a few days. We have short-lived bacteria that live for a few minutes to a few days and then more long-lived bacteria that can stay in our gut for years. If we switch to a healthier diet and change the other factors that affect gut health, such as exercise and stress, a whole new set of healthy bacteria can start to emerge, leading to improved health.

My Struggles with Constipation

We would consider it dog abuse to not feed our dogs healthy foods. Almost every dog owner knows the dangers of chocolate, grapes, and raisins for dogs. But many of us don't think twice about filling our own bodies with solely nutrient-poor or actively harmful substances. Sometimes, I want to shake my younger self to wake her up to this fact. But the older me has to be compassionate. I just didn't know what I didn't know.

I remember multiple visits to the emergency room with lower abdominal pain and chronic constipation. I saw numerous doctors and had imaging done. While everyone had an opinion, none of them suggested changing my diet. I then suffered through multiple disimpactions (removal of poop manually—not pleasant at all!) and had to undergo a diagnostic colonoscopy under anesthesia in my thirties. A gastroenterologist eventually diagnosed me with a motility disorder based on multiple sophisticated tests and prescribed fiber pills. I thought I had a physical problem with my gut, and I was doomed to take medication for the rest of my life. I begrudgingly accepted it was a disease I just had to deal with forever.

Many years later, once I started eating fruits and vegetables and cut out ultra-processed foods, my constipation magically disappeared. I started having a bowel movement every day. I didn't have a motility disorder—I had a "low fiber disorder!" Even though I didn't change my diet because of the constipation, I was thrilled. I was making these diet changes for other health reasons, specifically my high cholesterol, and resolving my constipation was a pleasant side effect. Win-win.

The Science of Fiber

Dietary fiber passes through the human gastrointestinal tract mostly intact, providing multiple health benefits along the way. Fiber can be classified into soluble and insoluble fiber.[326] Soluble fiber, when ingested, helps lower cholesterol and stabilizes our blood sugar levels. Soluble fiber includes fruits, lentils, beans, whole oats, and vegetables. Insoluble fiber adds bulk to stool because it doesn't dissolve in water. This is the type of fiber that helps us have regular bowel movements and prevents constipation. Insoluble fiber is found in whole grains, vegetables, and fruits (especially the skins of fruits).

The fiber associated with the natural sugars in fruits slows down the absorption of sugars into the blood, which helps in regulating our blood sugar (and avoiding the spikes seen when the fiber is missing).[327-329] One of the most common problems in our diet is juice. Juice naturally is calorie-dense, as seen in Figure 10.2. A tall glass of juice can be two hundred calories. In addition, because juice doesn't contain the fiber found in whole fruits, our body absorbs all its sugars into the bloodstream. While drinking juices is definitely better than sodas, it's best to avoid juices and instead eat whole fruits or use whole fruits in smoothies.

Cholesterol

Let's say it again: Plant-based whole foods have *minimal* cholesterol. Dietary cholesterol is mostly found in animal products, to the magnitude of "several hundreds to thousands fold" more than in plants.[330]

What is good about cholesterol? Cholesterol is a type of fat that is an essential part of every cell in our bodies. It's necessary for our cell membranes to keep fluids in and out. Cholesterol is also essential for the synthesis of certain hormones, like the stress hormone cortisol as well as the sex hormones testosterone and estrogen. And we need it to produce bile acid, which helps us digest foods, and for the conversion of vitamin D absorbed through the skin. Cholesterol is not a problem in itself—the problem lies in overconsumption and not having the benefit of fiber in our diet.[331] The cholesterol our bodies need is produced in our liver, and it's enough for us to function. We don't need additional cholesterol from our diet.

Unhealthy Fats

Though advertisers and lobbyists, some of whom partner with the U.S. government, would like you to think eggs are healthy, they are particularly rich in cholesterol.[332] All meats have cholesterol, including the often misleadingly labeled "white meats" (chicken and pork). Meat is meat. Dairy products, especially cheese, are another major source of cholesterol. Shellfish like shrimp and lobster can also be very high in dietary cholesterol.

Some animal products are even in medicines, cosmetics, and lotions.[333,334] That's why I've seen patients sometimes become allergic to certain medications. They may be sensitive to the animal products in the pill's capsule. Basically, the body sees these animal products as foreign objects and mounts an inflammatory response to them.

This section is not about discouraging you or overwhelming you. You don't have to do a complete turn-around and strictly eat vegetables. It's about giving you information so you can make a choice based on facts. I can offer a personal example here about the power of choices. Before I knew the downsides of animal-based foods, I used to eat two eggs with a large glass of juice many mornings, thinking it was healthy. I would eat meat products at every meal and make sure I had dairy twice a day. I was convinced what I was doing was healthy, but later, after facing my own health challenges and doing much research, I realized I had been misled. Now, I make different choices and minimize these unhealthy fats in my diet.

Carbs

In order to move and to survive, humans need carbs.

Carbs are short for carbohydrates. Foods are processed in different ways depending on their types (meats, vegetables, starches, dairy, etc.) through complex biochemical reactions into macronutrients within our digestive systems. Carbs are good for you as long as they're in the form of whole food or complex form. The refined and processed carbs are the problem because almost all the nutrients and beneficial fiber have been removed during processing.

If we eat zero carbs in our diet, the fat and protein we eat will be converted into carbs.[335,336] Eventually, the body moves to burning fat into ketone bodies, which can be used for energy through ketosis. This is an operating principle of the Keto diet, which is low in sugars and carbs and high in fats and proteins. It relies on the body's ability to transform fat and protein into carbs. But Keto diets can affect liver health and lead to nutritional deficiencies, especially since animal-based Keto diets lack dietary fiber.[337]

As stated before, animal-based foods do not contain fiber. These animal-based foods may also increase heart attack and stroke risks from the high levels of cholesterol, trans fats, and saturated fats. Many who follow the Keto diet over time metabolically adjust to the low carbohydrates and their metabolic rate decreases, making it hard to maintain weight loss.[338] In addition, eating too few carbohydrates is associated with as much of an increased risk of death from all causes as eating too many carbohydrates.[339]

Dairy

As humans, should we be drinking milk from other animal species? That is, should we continue to drink dairy cow milk in childhood and adulthood after breastfeeding is done in infancy? Many experts say "no." We don't need cow's milk for our health any more than we need dog milk or cat milk. I would suggest that humans are not *lactose intolerant*, but simply should not be drinking milk from any species except other humans—we are instead *milk-from-other species-intolerant*.

Cows must produce milk for their calves so they can grow exponentially fast. When we drink cow milk, we're taking in a lot of animal proteins we don't really need. Because cows in dairy farms are artificially made to produce milk year-round, many milk-producing cows develop mastitis, which produces pus in the milk.[340] In fact, globally, oversight bodies regulate how much bacteria and microorganisms are present in our milk. In the U.S., the Food and Drug Administration (FDA) limits how much pus can be in the cow's milk we buy from our grocery stores, but it is still there.[341] The pus and bovine animal proteins are foreign to our bodies, so when we consume milk, our bodies mount an inflammatory response, and they later develop the diagnosis of lactose intolerant. But, as I stated earlier, I don't believe in that diagnosis. I think, as humans, we are all *milk-from-other species-intolerant*.

For me, once I stopped consuming dairy all together, I went from a chronically stuffed up nose and allergies (requiring me to use a box or two of tissues per week to blow my nose, to now being almost completely allergy-free. I am happy to report that, currently, tissue boxes sit on my side tables long enough to collect dust before becoming empty.

Cheese

In Figure 10.2, cheese is depicted as one of the most calorie-dense foods, meaning it has a significant number of calories in a small portion. It's high in saturated fats and leads to elevations of LDL cholesterol, otherwise known as the "bad" cholesterol. Many cheeses also have high salt content and additives.

Those of us living in European countries eat cheese regularly, but not in the bulk and quantity we do in the U.S. In the U.S., we currently consume about 40 pounds of cheese per person per year. Just a few decades ago in the 1970s, we were consuming only 12 pounds per person.[342] That's a huge increase.

Some physicians, like Neal Barnard of the Physicians Committee for Responsible Medicine, have studied this issue in depth.[343] The increase in cheese consumption is correlated to negative biological consequences—while we can't prove causation, it's worth considering. Certain chemicals in cheese are very addictive, called *casomorphins*. Casomorphins have opioid-like properties in the brain and interact with the same pleasure and reward receptors in the brain that opioids do.[344] Also, research suggests cheese may increase dopamine in our bodies because of the high fat content, leading many people to crave the dopamine rush.[345]

While many good books have been written about nutrition and this chapter could be much longer, I hope the discussion helps set the stage for changes. Please see my website www.giamerlo.com for resources.

Other important aspects of nutrients and their consumption to consider when making dietary changes are ever so briefly summarized in the following sections.

Sugar

In a whole fruit, the naturally occurring sugars are bound to fiber and contain healthy phytonutrients. This fiber regulates how our bodies process the sugar.[346] As described earlier, whole fruits don't cause the same spikes in blood sugar. Therefore, the sugar in fruits needs to be consumed with the whole fruit, not as juices where the fiber is all removed.

Sugars present one of the biggest dangers in our diet. Sugar addiction is discussed in more detail in Chapter 15: Substance Use Harm Reduction.

Oil

Everybody knows we shouldn't put oil down our kitchen pipes—the same is true for our bodies. Dietary oil can clog our arteries, elevate cholesterol levels, introduce trans fats into our bodies, and predispose us to strokes and heart attacks.[347] This dietary oil includes oil in our fried foods, cooking oil, and other added oils in foods. Additionally, there is a body of research suggesting that some olive oils have pesticides and as such may be endocrine disruptors.[348,349]

Other research has suggested that extra-virgin olive oil contains healthy antioxidants called polyphenols.[350] With all the potential negative effects of oils in the body, I would suggest minimizing the amount you consume. Many other sources exist for healthy antioxidant polyphenols including flaxseeds, chestnuts, hazelnuts, pecans, almonds, and many fruits and vegetables.[351]

It is possible to cook healthy, tasty, whole food, plant-based meals without, or with minimum amounts of sugar, oil, or salt. ChefAJ at www.ChefAJ.com is an excellent resource for cooking without and/or minimizing sugar, oil, or salt (also called *SOS-free* cooking).

Salt/Sodium

Too much salt will overburden our kidneys, causing high blood pressure, otherwise known as hypertension. A not-too-uncommon malady I see is too little sodium caused by drinking too much water. As described before, both ends of the spectrum—dehydration and overhydration—can be problematic.

Salt is often used as a preservative in processed foods, and this is especially true for ultra-processed foods.

Foods for Brain Health

While much is known about the health benefits of certain foods for physical health, the area of nutritional psychiatry is an emerging field. Nutritional psychiatry, a subfield of lifestyle psychiatry, discusses the foods that may be helpful for brain health, including alleviating some mental health symptoms. While it is an emerging field, there are some general guidelines that may be helpful. Please review Table 10.1 for a list of brain-healthy foods. As always, make sure these are consumed in moderation and after discussing with your physician, especially turmeric as it may lead to unexpected complications.

Table 10.1 Eight Powerful Brain Health Foods

Food	Brain Response
Green, Leafy Vegetables	Kale, spinach, and collard greens may slow cognitive decline. Limit consumption of spinach as the oxalates may cause kidney problems.
Berries	Blueberries, strawberries, blackberries, etc., all contain significant flavonoids (e.g., anthocyanins) that may improve memory and delay memory decline. Blueberries, especially, may be considered a superfood for brain health.
Nuts	Walnuts and almonds, which contain high levels of omega-3 and alpha-linolenic acid (ALA), are especially helpful for improved cognition, including memory. However, as they are highly caloric, nuts should be consumed in moderation.
Dark Chocolate	Dark chocolate contains flavonoids, which may increase blood flow to the brain. Aim to eat only non-dairy dark chocolate, as the dairy may interfere with this function.
Cruciferous vegetables	Broccoli, cauliflower, bok choy, brussels sprouts, cabbage, and other cruciferous vegetables may help prevent dementia through a compound called sulforaphane. Through other mechanisms they preserve brain health.
Fruits	Citrus fruits and other foods high in vitamin C (tomatoes, kiwi, raw bell pepper) may prevent mental decline, and through their antioxidant effects, reduce free radical formation. Fruits may also decrease blood pressure and high cholesterol, thereby preventing strokes in the brain.
Turmeric	Turmeric is best consumed in foods and not as a pill—too much can be detrimental. Curcumin, the active ingredient in turmeric, is a potent antioxidant and anti-inflammatory that may help improve memory, improve depression, and slow age-related decline. Fruits may also decrease blood pressure and high cholesterol, thereby preventing strokes in the brain.
Green Tea	Green tea may improve alertness, memory, focus, and support brain health. They are also rich in antioxidants and polyphenols, which reduce the risk of mental decline.

Conclusion

There are many competing and conflicting sources of information suggesting what is healthy and unhealthy for us to eat. What is clear, however, is that we continue to have an epidemic of man-made, noncommunicable chronic diseases worldwide. The foods we eat have changed dramatically over the last few decades, and the science of food has evolved. Arguments on both sides of the table will always exist about what is fact or fiction regarding food. I strongly suggest not worrying about the politics of this polarized conversation. Instead, focus on the aspects we can change for our personal and our family's health.

Some things cannot be refuted: ultra-processed foods are unhealthy, inflammation is wreaking havoc onto our bodies, the standard American diet is indeed SAD, and—when used properly—food can be medicine and heal us.

Reducing our consumption of ultra-processed foods is important in the process of *Restack*-ing our blocks. We and our gut microbiota need healthy foods. Though it can be somewhat gross to think about the gut microbiota inside of us, these organisms are what keep us nourished and healthy. While we cannot change many things in the world, we can be empowered by viewing our body as a temple and treating it with kindness and respect.

Chapter 11: Restorative Sleep

We spend 20 to 35 years of our lives sleeping.

Of course, that's for the fortunate of us who live to an old age. Generally, we spend a third of our lives sleeping. It bears repeating because it shows just how much our bodies need sleep. Many Americans are getting less than the required sleep per night—seven hours of sleep is needed to prevent disease and promote health. In this chapter, we will discuss what sleep is and how it's measured. We will then focus on some of the *Restack*-ing techniques for preventing and treating disorders of sleep.

Sleep can best be defined as a state where we're cut off from our external environment and outside stimulation.[352] When we're asleep, our bodies are still going through numerous internal changes and activities. Our bodies use this time for physical and mental restoration and to consolidate our memories from the day. Our immune function becomes regulated and important hormones are produced. Sleep is essential to many of our body's vital and emotional functions, so inadequate or low-quality sleep can lead to irritability, moodiness, and the breakdown of essential bodily functions. On the flip side, reintegrating healthy sleep patterns into our lives may help *Restack* us by improving our mood, decreasing our irritability, and promoting healthy bodily functions.

Before reading this chapter, reflect on your sleep patterns in Rx 11.1. This chapter will address the questions in the Rx, and your answers can point you in the direction of interventions to improve your sleep.

R̶X 11.1 Reflecting on Your Sleep Patterns
Prescription

1. How many hours do you sleep per night? Too much or too little sleep might be something you want to address.

2. How many minutes does it take you to fall asleep at night? Difficulty falling asleep can be helped with improved sleep hygiene, which will be discussed in Rx 11.2.

3. Do you wake up in the middle of the night and are unable to fall back asleep? Waking up to use the restroom doesn't count, as long as you're able to fall back asleep after.

4. Do you feel tired during the day? Getting adequate sleep at night and sleep hygiene are important.

5. Do you have any physical or mental health conditions? Certain conditions may be related to sleep difficulties.

Why Do We Need Sleep?

The cells in our body each have their own cycles from birth to death. Some cells last a month. Some cells last a year. Our cells must follow their natural cycles to function properly, and much of this cycle happens while we're asleep. As we're resting, our bodies are repairing our cells' DNA and detoxifying our systems.[353] Without these repair stages, we can experience disruptions in our brain health. Thus, it's crucial we get enough sleep, that our sleep is of good quality, and it happens on a regular schedule.

Worldwide, about 20% of workers are on the night shift.[354] Our current global economy—requiring us to access goods 24/7—requires people to work night shifts. Suddenly starting a night shift can throw our circadian rhythm off balance, leading to an increased risk of insomnia. But the economic benefit must also be balanced with the fact that insomnia directly represents $94.9 billion in healthcare costs annually.[355] Indirect costs from insomnia, through causes such as loss of productivity at work, workplace injuries, and motor vehicle accidents, may be in excess of one trillion dollars annually.[355]

Table 11.1 Sleep and Chronic Diseases[356-366]	
Chronic Disease	Effects of Sleep Deprivation on Disease
Type 2 Diabetes	Sleep deprivation can affect glucose metabolism and insulin sensitivity.
Obesity	Poor sleep has been noted to be associated with weight gain and obesity through many mechanisms, most notably, disturbed sleep affects hunger hormones that lead to increased appetite and subsequent overeating.
Cancer	There are studies that connect poor sleep with an increased risk of breast and prostate cancers.
COPD	The severity of respiratory disorders and lung functioning is worsened with sleep disturbances.
Cognitive disorders	Individuals with disturbed sleep are at greater risk of developing cognitive decline and Alzheimer's.
Mood and mental health disorders	Sleep deprivation is associated with poor frustration tolerance, irritability, and increased risk of suicide (described in detail in Table 11.2).

Moreover, what is the cost to our bodies? Lack of sleep is specifically linked to numerous chronic diseases as summarized in Table 11.1.[356-366]

A Case of Sleep and Mental Health Conditions

In my practice, when I address lifestyle with patients, I usually start with the pillar on restorative sleep because it's often the intervention that can make the biggest impact. One case involved Jamie, a 30-year-old graduate student who came to me for treatment for extreme anxiety symptoms, which she had been attempting to control with benzodiazepines, commonly called benzos. Upon evaluation, I noted she was only getting two to three hours of sleep per night. Over the next few months, Jamie was able to follow a plan to sleep and wake up at regular times. She darkened her bedroom so the lights didn't wake her up, decreased drinking liquids a few hours before sleep so she didn't wake up in the middle of the night, and stopped taking her laptop to bed so the blue lights didn't affect her sleep. These sleep interventions helped her so much that she no longer relied on benzos and was able to stop taking them. She had experienced her symptoms as anxiety, for which she had been prescribed the medication. However, the root cause was the quality and quantity of her sleep, not anxiety. For some patients, they may still have anxiety after their sleep is regulated, but they find the anxiety better and they need less medication to manage it.

A bidirectional relationship exists between mental health and sleep. This is true for many mental health conditions, which are summarized in Table 11.2.[367-382]

Overall, we need sleep for our cognition as well as to help us regulate our moods, concentrate, cope with stress, and make decisions. Numerous studies show that people with poor sleep habits have an increased risk of all-cause mortality, which means death due to any cause whether it's related to a physical or mental health condition or not.[383]

Consequences of Sleep Deprivation

The consequences of sleep deprivation can be dramatic in extreme cases. For example, throughout history, prisoners of war have often been tortured through sleep deprivation. After three days of no sleep, thoughts become disordered, and someone may become paranoid or experience visual and auditory hallucinations. After a week, confusion may worsen, and the individual may experience psychotic thinking. Ultimately, the immune system becomes weakened with prolonged sleep deprivation. Potentially life-threatening physical health issues like heart problems and metabolic disturbances may develop.[384]

Table 11.2 Sleep and Mental Health Conditions[367-382]	
Mental Health Condition	Relationship Between Sleep Deprivation and Mental Health Condition
Depression	Sleep disturbances are common, especially early morning waking, insomnia, or sometimes oversleeping. Also, not getting enough sleep over long periods of time can increase your risk of developing depression.
Suicidal thoughts	In those with suicidal ideation, poor sleep may be associated with the feeling of hopelessness.
Bipolar disorder	During the manic phase, there is a reduced need for sleep, and while in the depressive phase, there may be excessive sleep.
Anxiety disorders	Sleep can be impaired with difficulty falling and staying asleep. And, if you don't get enough sleep, your feelings of anxiety can worsen.
Posttraumatic stress disorder (PTSD)	Sleep problems include nightmares, insomnia, and fragmented sleep, all of which are often related to the traumatic event.

"Sleep Is for Babies" Fallacy

When I was growing up, one of the most commonly uttered things I heard around my friends during sleepovers was, "Sleep is for babies." Many of my friends from middle school would think it was cool to stay up late and, chronically, not get enough sleep at night. During high school, many of my friends were overloaded with advanced placement classes, requiring four to six hours of homework on a regular school night and much more during exam season. This is when most kids in the 1980s started drinking coffee. Now, of course, one of the biggest problems I see is kids overusing energy drinks and the explosion of the use of Adderall and other stimulants to help them stay awake and focus better on schoolwork. The downplaying of the importance of sleep grew worse in medical school when I and many of my colleagues were chronically sleep deprived. The general atmosphere was one of *bravado* associated with not needing sleep, or being able to "suck it up" and stay awake all night.

FIGURE 11.1 STAGES OF SLEEP [387]

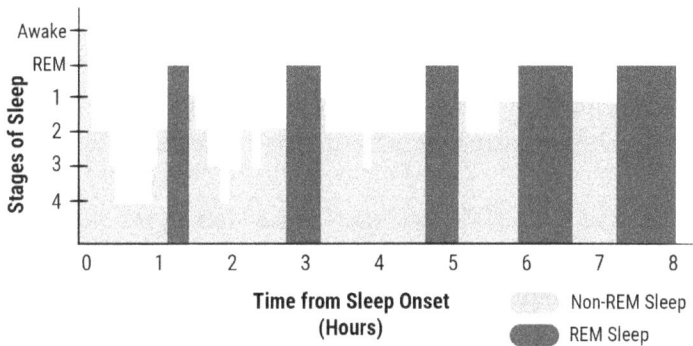

Too Much Sleep

On the other hand, oversleeping can be just as dangerous to your health. Similar to sleep deprivation, consistently sleeping more than 10 hours per night has also been associated with global cognitive decline.[385] Long-duration sleep has been linked to memory impairments in older adults, though the mechanism has not been completely worked out by researchers. Some theories include brain changes, such as thinning of the cortex in the frontal temporal areas or inflammatory pathways with interleukin-6 (IL-6) and C-reactive protein (CRP). Additionally, chronically oversleeping is also associated with heart disease and obesity.[386]

Sleep Stages and Duration

What does good sleep look like?

To understand how to manage our sleep in a healthy manner, we first must understand some of the basic science behind the sleep cycle. Figure 11.1 shows the four stages of sleep.[387] Understanding the purpose of each of these sleep stages is essential for those of us who don't get enough sleep or get too much sleep. Stages 1 and 2, the lighter stages of sleep, are useful in preparing us for stages 3 and 4, where the body's restorative work, such as cellular repair, occurs.

Note that most of the REM sleep takes place later in the sleep cycle. So, for those of us sleeping six hours or less, what are the consequences? Well, we're missing out on principal functions of REM sleep, which is needed to help restore cognition, consolidate memories, and aid us in learning and processing our emotions.

How Much Do We Need to Sleep Across Our Lifespan?

Given what we know about the sleep cycle, a certain duration of sleep is recommended to benefit from the vital restorative role of REM sleep. Figure 11.2 illustrates that the duration of sleep needed varies across the lifespan.[388] For example, we recommend that newborns have 14 to 17 hours asleep, infants have 12 to 15, and adults need about 7 to 9 hours of sleep. It should be noted that pregnant women need a different duration of sleep given the fragmentation of sleep they may experience in the second and third trimesters.[389]

But other factors are also important beyond sleep duration, like sleep timing and consistency. Many studies show that the healthiest patterns involve going to sleep earlier in the night, sleeping according to the same bedtime and wake-up times, and "catching up" on sleep on the weekends as needed.[388]

FIGURE 11.2 RECOMMENDED SLEEP DURATION FOR DIFFERENT AGE GROUPS [386]

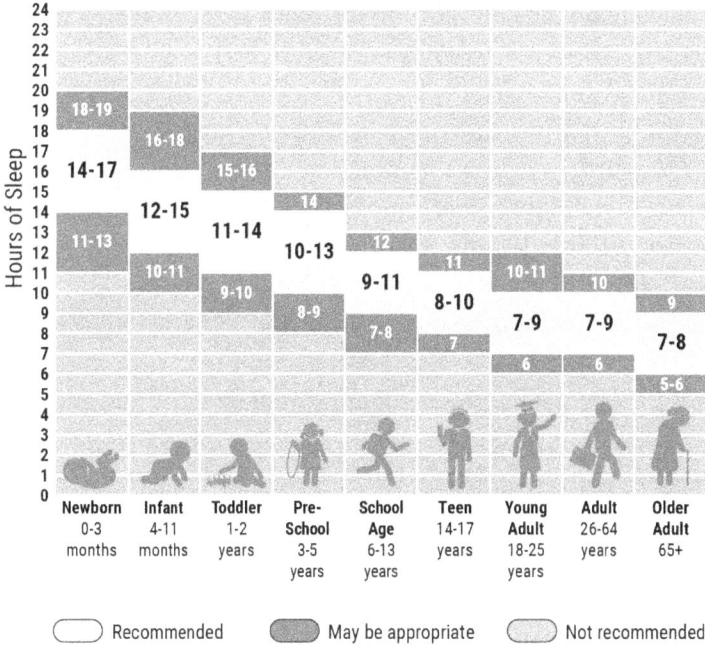

Adapted from Max Hirshkowitz, Kaitlyn Whiton, Steven M. Albert, Cathy Alessi, Oliviero Bruni, Lydia DonCarlos, Nancy Hazen, John Herman, Paula J. Adams Hillard, Eliot S. Katz, et al., "National Sleep Foundation's Updated Sleep Duration Recommendations: Final Report," Sleep Health 1, no. 4 (2015): 233–243

The Internal Clock and Sleep Timing

What we call our "internal clock" is the *circadian rhythm*, which regulates our bodies on an approximately 24-hour cycle. The circadian rhythm is regulated by the hypothalamus, which is in a similar area to the brain regions regulating serotonin for mood, norepinephrine for alertness, and trauma activation.[390] This interconnectedness helps explain how vital bodily functions, among other things, are so highly impacted by restorative or unhealthy sleep. Our circadian rhythm is also determined by external stimuli, particularly light and darkness.

This internal clock alerts us at about 9 am and decreases until 9 pm with the greatest feeling of alertness occurring early in the morning.[390] One of the keys to healthy sleep is to work with this schedule rather than against it. This means avoiding habits that will make us artificially alert when our body wants to wind down, or artificially sluggish when our body wants to wake up. It involves combating psychological arousal, often called the "fight-or-flight" syndrome, which is associated with alertness and preparing us for action. If we experience "fight-or-flight" while sleeping, our sleep can become fragmented and shallow as we're no longer able to cut off from monitoring what's happening externally, that is, outside our sleeping bodies. The need to monitor what is happening externally is part of the "fight-or-flight" response to defend ourselves in situations of danger.

Psychological arousal is regulated by the reticular activating system in the brain which keeps us active during the day but prohibits sleep when stimulated.[391] The reticular activating system is affected by muscle tension, pain, and stress hormones. To get adequate and restful sleep, we need to have a minimal amount of muscle tension, a minimal amount of pain, and decreased stress hormones.

What are Sleep Hygiene Techniques?

Behavioral and environmental recommendations to foster restorative sleep can be generalized to most people in most situations.[392,393] These are often referred to as "sleep hygiene techniques." Review Rx 11.2, which lists techniques and recommendations for improving your sleep hygiene.

242

Sleep Relaxation Techniques

Relaxing requires shutting off our brains and enjoying calm ways to minimize our thinking about the external world. In addition to sleep hygiene techniques, it may be helpful to use techniques to help prepare us for sleep.

Some sleep relaxation techniques include:
1. Diaphragmatic breathing and meditation.
2. Progressive meditation or imagining positive scenarios.
3. Engaging in enjoyable, relaxing things before sleeping like taking a bath.
4. Keeping a gratitude journal or journaling our worries on a piece of paper so we can lay them aside.

Sleep and CBT

It may be helpful to approach changing your sleep habits in a systematic manner, the way we might do in cognitive behavioral therapy (CBT).[394] While CBT is a manualized, evidence-based treatment that needs to be performed by a trained clinician, we can employ some of the techniques with a self-help approach. In the self-help approach, we reflect on our thoughts and behavioral processes in a systematic way. This can then help us change our approach, remove blocks for healthy sleep, and *Restack* ourselves. Using Rx 11.3, you can attempt this process for yourself.

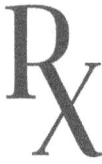

R⨯ 11.2 Sleep Hygiene Techniques and Recommendations
Prescription

1. **Liquids:** Avoid consuming excessive liquids before going to bed.

2. **Meals:** Eat on a consistent schedule during the day and early evening. Don't skip meals. Circadian rhythm is affected by eating, so if you don't eat consistently during the day, it will interfere with your sleep.

3. **Sunlight:** Expose yourself to as much sunlight as possible early in the day and as little sunlight and artificial light in the evening. This is because light inhibits melatonin production and tells the body that it needs to stay awake.

4. **Exercise:** Exercise regularly during the day. However, avoid exercise within four hours of bedtime because exercise raises your core body temperature, making you feel more alert.

5. **Caffeine and other stimulants:** Don't drink caffeine or any other energizing substance after five o'clock in the evening.

6. **Alcohol:** Limit alcohol intake. Alcohol can impair your sleep cycle, leading to difficulty in maintaining a consistent schedule. You may initially feel more sleepy after drinking alcohol, but alcohol disrupts and decreases REM sleep, leading to cognitive impairment and mood disturbances. Alcohol is also associated with relaxing the muscles in the throat, worsening snoring and sleep apnea in those who have these conditions.

7. **Tobacco:** Limit tobacco intake.

8. **Napping:** Avoid daytime naps longer than 20 minutes.

9. **Stress management:** Manage your worries and anxieties. Sometimes, this means avoiding thoughts about your losses or fears and what's going on in life. These thoughts can make it very difficult to sleep because they prompt worry, which is a manifestation of stress.

10. **Distractions:** Minimize noise in the bedroom.

11. **A bed is for sleep:** Avoid using the bed for things other than sleep. This helps your brain associate your bed with sleep time.

12. **Minimizing blue light:** Minimize screen use in the bedroom, including smart-phones, iPads, TVs, or computers.

13. **Medications:** Many medications also impair sleep, so discuss potential side effects with your doctor. The list is long and includes many over-the-counter medications like decongestants and pain medications.

R̶X̶ 11.3 Changing Your Sleep Habits
Prescription

1. Review Tables 11.1 and 11.2. Make note of any of the physical or psychiatric disorders you may have which may be affecting your sleep.

2. Assess your sleep habits by reviewing Figures 11.1 and 11.2. Are you satisfied with your sleeping patterns? Are you getting enough sleep?

3. Review the sleep hygiene techniques in Rx 11.2 and the sleep relaxation techniques discussed earlier in this chapter. Brainstorm possible changes that you can make to improve the quality of your sleep.

4. Look at the barriers that you may have in employing these techniques. Is there a way to cognitively restructure your relationship with some of your lifestyle practices, through Rx 5.1 The Thought Ladder and Action Roof Exercise? Think of strategies that can address these barriers. Pay particular attention to how the sleep-wake cycle (that is, the circadian rhythm) is affected by your lifestyle.

5. Finally, employ interventions like changing your sleep hygiene habits, using cognitive restructuring through relaxation techniques, and limiting potential barriers in your environment.

Assistive Technology

As we discussed earlier, the first step to regulating our sleep is to measure and evaluate it. We can use a number of tools to do that.

Mobile devices are used quite frequently now to assess our sleep but should be used with caution as the reliability and accuracy of the gathered data can be questionable. Examples include ActiGraph wearable devices, wireless electroencephalograms (EEGs), smartwatches/fitness trackers/mobile phone sensing, and ultrasound sensors.[395-397]

Self-Reported Questionnaires

In this chapter, we have covered a lot of ground about sleep. If you find your symptoms are severe or you can't get a handle on sleep even with the self-help practices, you may benefit from seeing a sleep specialist. The specialist may suggest a formal evaluation, which may include a sleep study.

A physician may use additional formalized questionnaires in clinical practice. Two often-used questionnaires include the PSQI and the ESS:

- *Pittsburgh Sleep Quality Index* (PSQI) looks at the quality of sleep over one month and grades on 19 individual items and 7 components.[398]
- The *Epworth Sleepiness Scale*(ESS) is a quick scale that can help diagnose clinical sleep disorders.[399]

Sleep Is the Backbone of Our Health

Sleep encompasses multiple facets, not simply how much sleep we're getting, but the quality of our sleep and our sleep environment. Since sleep is so important, reflecting on our sleep patterns can be helpful in improving our everyday health and *Restack*-ing ourselves. Sleep is connected to many chronic diseases, both mental and physical. Sometimes we can improve sleep using self-help techniques, though sometimes, we may need to seek expert care. In lifestyle psychiatry, addressing sleep can often improve depression, anxiety, and other mental health disorders. For good reason, sleep is one of the six pillars of lifestyle psychiatry.

And, no, sleep is *not* just for babies.

Chapter 12: Physical Activity and Movement

Mark thought his life might be coming to an end. I had treated him 20 years before for depression, and he came back, now an 82-year-old retired male who was having issues remembering things and feeling "blah." He couldn't pinpoint a reason to continue to live but denied any suicidal thoughts. He said his mood was "okay," but then talked about not finding pleasure in many things anymore. His primary care physician referred him to me with a question of him being clinically depressed.

He said, "But that's just old age, right, Doc?" He appeared healthy and was cleared for all sorts of exercise by his doctor. However, he hesitated. "I stopped going on walks when my wife died 10 years ago. I don't know, Doc, that was something we enjoyed doing together. It just doesn't feel right." He then told me his family was worried about his memory, but he remarked, "I'm fine. I'm 82, you know? What can you expect?"

We talked about things he enjoyed in the past including spending time with grandkids, having lunch with friends at the diner, watching old movies, and keeping up with his favorite sports teams. Though he had lost some interest in these things, he was able to verbalize his "why" and started embracing the potential to enjoy himself again. Because walks were maybe too triggering for him after the loss of his wife, I suggested he try a treadmill. He shrugged his shoulders and said, "Okay, why not?"

We worked to slowly increase his time and speed on the treadmill, from slow walking to power walking. Over the course of six months, his mood improved, his cognitive abilities and memory got better, and he started making friends with people at the gym.

At eight months, he came to me with a gleam in his eyes. "Maybe walking outside isn't a bad idea after all." He exuded hope and began to enjoy his life again.

Why Do We Need Movement?

In the physical health world, many experts are now shying away from the terms "exercise" and "physical activity" and focusing on "movement." Movement allows inclusion for those of us who need to have less intense regimens because of age, physical mobility issues, sedentary lifestyles, preferences, or doctors' advice cautioning physical activity because of medical issues. For the purposes of this chapter, please use the definition that works better for you. Much of the research to date has focused on the terms "exercise" and "physical activity," and therefore, I will more often than not use those terms.

Physical activity not only supports physical health, but also has a serious and profound effect on mental health. For our physical health, it reduces the potential of developing diseases like cancer, heart disease, diabetes, and dementia. In fact, our risk of death from *any* cause is decreased by up to 33% with regular physical exercise.[400]

For our mental health, we have a 47% greater likelihood of struggling with depression if we have poor fitness.[401] We can improve our thinking and delay the risk of dementia and other forms of cognitive decline with regular exercise, which we will discuss in detail later in this chapter.

Being physically active can affect both mental and physical health in numerous ways. Table 12.1 describes the benefit of physical activity on multiple aspects of health, including brain health, heart health, bone health, metabolic health, cancer avoidance, and overall health.[402-404]

Table 12.1 Physical Activity on Physical and Mental Health[402-404]

Body Systems	Outcome
Brain Health (Mental Health and Cognition):	
– Depression and depressed mood	Reduced risk of depression and depressed mood
– Anxiety	Reduced immediate and long-term feelings of anxiety
– Stress	Reduced stress and acute stress response
– Cognition (and Dementia)	Children (ages 6-13): Improved performance on academic achievement tests, memory, executive function, and processing speed Adults: Reduced risk of dementia (including Alzheimer's disease) Adults (age > 50): Improved executive function, attention, memory, and processing speed
– Schizophrenia	May diminish schizophrenia symptom frequency and severity
– Bipolar disorder	Associated with decreased depressive symptoms and improved quality of life and functioning
Heart Health	Reduced risk of hypertension, coronary artery disease, heart failure, and stroke
Bone Health	Improved bone health, reduced risk of osteoporosis, and reduced risk of fracture
Metabolic Health	Reduced risk and helps control type 2 diabetes, obesity, and poor lipid levels
Cancer	Reduced risk of bladder, breast, colon, endometrial, esophageal, kidney, lung, and stomach cancer
General Health	Improved sleep quality, decreased stress, and reduced risk of chronic fatigue

We need movement not only for our individual health, but also for preventative reasons. We spend so much money globally on healthcare for chronic diseases, which could be prevented if we all moved more. The cost associated with lack of physical activity in the U.S. is estimated at about $120 billion annually.[405]

A Case of Physical Activity and Improved Mental Health

Jack, a 19-year-old college student studying engineering reported a long history of "feeling irritated all the time." He said that he thinks that it's due to his course of study that he really liked when he started, but now unsure because he cannot feel inspired to read a single textbook. He feels like a failure and has no energy, and Jack reported countless nights of waking up in the middle of the night and not being able to go back to sleep. He felt like he lost pleasure in doing things, and said, "Well, what's the point? I can't focus enough to study anyway." He denied having thoughts of hurting others or himself, and denied hearing voices or seeing things. Jack never had a history of depression or any suicidal risk factors. He was resistant to medication, and after a thorough evaluation, appeared to have a diagnosis of mild to moderate depression. After assessing his lifestyle vital signs (diet, physical activity, sleep, stress management, connectedness, and substance use similar to the self-assessment Rx 2.1), he and I had a discussion about which one of the lifestyle factors concerns him the most. He said that, even though he has trouble sleeping at night, he thinks that his bigger issue is that he has put on 40 pounds over the last few years, consequently limiting his social activity and confidence. He also agreed that his energy may be affected by his lack of physical activity.

Jack talked about the painful breakup with his only girlfriend that he had since he was 15, and the pressure that he feels to do well in school since his family is counting on him to be successful, as he is the first member of his family to go to college. He said, "Going back home is stressful because all they can focus on is how easy their life will be once I graduate and can take care of everybody." He's been to enough lectures about career planning to know that his job outside of college is going to be a lot more than his family had, but may not be enough to give them the life of luxury they imagine. As we started planning a physical activity goal, I referred him to his college clinic, and he was cleared for an exercise routine.

Using the *Restack Model of Change*, we settled upon a routine of Jack walking to the school gym, which was six blocks away, every day for the next two weeks. He did not have to enter, but rather he was simply instructed to walk there and go back home. That alleviated a lot of his stress around his exercise anxiety and made him feel accomplished in following the routine. This goal may have seemed easy for most, but was challenging for Jack since he would rarely leave his dorm room except to go downstairs to the dining hall. After two weeks, he came back to my office, proud of himself, and showed me the steps that he had walked on his phone–it was a progression from his former negligible steps per day to thousands now. We then planned for him to do this twice a week, and ultimately, three times a week while still not setting forth inside the gym. Ultimately, he jogged back and forth three times every time he went there. A month and a half later, he came to my office, said his sleep had improved, and explained excitedly that he was looking at his college's amateur band so that he could go and play the trumpet. He used to be really good at it in high school, and it brought him joy. Jack also remarked that one time when he was jogging to the gym, he met one of his classmates and they both jogged to a local diner to eat dinner together.

Jack then said to me, "I think I'm ready to start exercising. What do you think, Doc?" I reinforced the physical movement that he'd been doing, which was also equally important as formal exercise in the gym. Over the next few months, I supported his desire to incorporate strength training and, ultimately, cardio into his daily routine. Jack's mood continued to improve, he had a newfound pleasure in playing the trumpet, and he started making friends for the first time in college.

What are the Components of Physical Activity?

Physical activity and movement can be broken down into five components, which include (1) cardio, (2) strength training, (3) flexibility, (4) balance, and (5) speed.[405]

"I take medications for my heart, Doc. I don't need to exercise."

So much misinformation about our health has been disseminated, especially about heart health. While we should always talk to our doctors about starting a movement program, medication doesn't solve or mitigate our need to move, exercise, or be active. "Cardio" is what we normally hear, which is short for "cardiovascular training" or "cardiopulmonary training" (both mean about the same thing). Cardio is also sometimes referred to as "aerobic activity."

1. Cardio (Cardiovascular Training)

Cardio is a workout for our heart, and it is individualized. For example, I would never recommend running a marathon to someone who has limited physical activity in their day-to-day. We have to train our hearts slowly and gradually to handle that level of activity. I have heard many horror stories in the winter of people having heart attacks after shoveling snow. Shoveling snow is a vigorous cardio activity, and your heart needs to be trained and ready for that. Someone can't go from "couch potato" to shoveling snow, just like someone can't go from "couch potato" to running a marathon. These are similar mistakes that can be life-threatening!

Levels of Cardio

Regular physical activity can be described as light, moderate, or vigorous. For physical activity to be helpful for our heart health, it doesn't mean we need to start vigorously, but we do need to plan to build up intensity to sufficiently exercise our hearts. Even with that said, moderate physical activity may be the goal for many of us. In fact, light activity is still good for our health (more on this later), but it may not be as beneficial for our hearts.

Remember, we all have to start somewhere. Let's not shame ourselves. Instead, let's pat ourselves on the back for taking the first step! And remember, something is always better than nothing, so please, do continue to move. It is benefiting you! I would suggest considering fun activities like dancing, hiking, skating, biking, swimming, and tennis as examples of cardio activities.

METs

What do we mean by moderate and vigorous physical activity? I want to introduce some terms that will help us pull the research data together. *Cardiorespiratory fitness* (CRF) is measured according to a concept called the *metabolic equivalent of tasks* (METs). Technically, one MET is equal to 3.5 milliliters of oxygen per kilogram per minute.[406]

Every moderate or vigorous activity we undertake has a MET associated with it. I will discuss this in greater depth shortly, but it's important to understand that if you and a workout partner are doing the same activity at the same intensity, you may have different METs because this measurement is based on your *individual* cardiac conditioning. When someone tells you a given activity can burn X number of calories, this isn't correct. Rather, it's based on an average that may not be accurate for a given individual. The number of calories you burn is impacted by a range of factors that are distinct for everyone. But ultimately, hanging in there and doing regular physical activity has a host of benefits for our heart and mental health, as depicted in Figure 12.1.[407]

FIGURE 12.1 BENEFITS OF REGULAR PHYSICAL ACTIVITY ON HEART HEALTH [407]

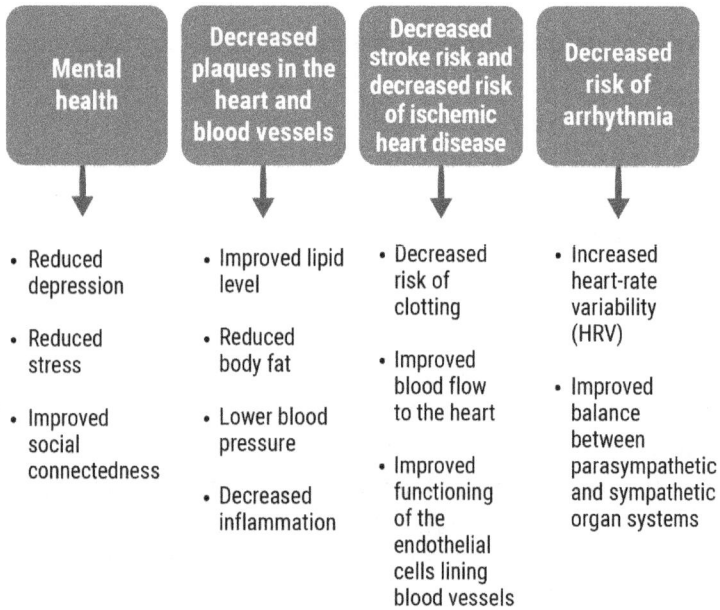

Mental health	Decreased plaques in the heart and blood vessels	Decreased stroke risk and decreased risk of ischemic heart disease	Decreased risk of arrhythmia
• Reduced depression • Reduced stress • Improved social connectedness	• Improved lipid level • Reduced body fat • Lower blood pressure • Decreased inflammation	• Decreased risk of clotting • Improved blood flow to the heart • Improved functioning of the endothelial cells lining blood vessels	• Increased heart-rate variability (HRV) • Improved balance between parasympathetic and sympathetic organ systems

We all have a resting metabolic rate for our level of exertion when we aren't doing physical activity. As we start performing moderate to vigorous physical activity, our need for oxygen to fuel our muscles increases, which increases this metabolic rate. The better our cardiovascular fitness, the less oxygen we will need because our hearts have adapted and become more efficient in using oxygen.

One MET is our resting metabolic rate, and 2 to 3 METs is our walking pace (considered a "light" activity). Faster walking is 3 to 5 METs, considered "moderate" activity, while jogging or running are 8 to 10 or more METs. Once again, this could change based on someone's heart health. For some people, jogging is a moderate activity because they're very conditioned. For others, walking may be a moderate or vigorous activity. Table 12.2 lists the METs of common physical activities.[408]

Table 12.2. Levels of Intensity of Common Activities in Metabolic Equivalent of Tasks (METs)[408]		
Light (<3.0 METs)	Moderate (3 - 5.9 METs)	Vigorous (≥6 METs)
Walking at a slow or leisurely pace (2 miles per hour or less)	Walking briskly (2.5 to 4 miles per hour)	Jogging or running
Cooking	Playing doubles tennis	Carrying heavy groceries
Light household chores	Raking the yard	Shoveling snow
Golfing	Mowing the lawn	Strenuous fitness class

An easy way to calculate your individual MET is by multiplying six times the heart rate index minus five. The formula is as follows:[409]

METs = (6 x Heart Rate Index) – 5

The *heart rate index* is your activity heart rate divided by your resting heart rate.

Let's explore how these two concepts relate to one another with some actual numbers. Let's say I have a resting heart rate of 60 beats per minute (bpm). That means, when I am sitting still and relaxing, my heart rate is about 60 bpm. When I attend my Orangetheory Fitness® session, my heart rate increases to 150 bpm. My heart rate index would be 150 divided by 60, which is 2.5. If I multiply this by 6, it equals 15. Then, that minus 5 equals 10 METs. So, my MET during my fitness class is 10, which is a vigorous activity for me—and for most people in that fitness class! But we all have different numbers when calculating our individual METs.

Heart Rate Variability

METs are not the end of the conversation. *Heart rate variability* (HRV) is also important for our cardiac health. HRV measures the difference in the times between our heartbeats in milliseconds. Sometimes, your heart may beat every 1.0 seconds or 1.4 seconds or 0.9 seconds. HRV varies by age, physical fitness, and day to day. It's related to our parasympathetic or sympathetic nervous system. Over time, our HRV changes. For those who have a health app on their smartphones, you can find a calculation of your HRV. Overall, a higher HRV is better than a lower one for your age group, indicating a dominance of the parasympathetic nervous system when the body is in relaxation mode. A lot of research shows this is a good measure to gauge our heart health, including our fitness level, stress levels, and other lifestyle pillars such as the quality of our sleep, diet, and alcohol intake.[410,411]

How Much Exercise Is Enough?

Why is cardio important, and how much should we be getting? The U.S. government, and many other countries, have developed physical activity guidelines. The recommendation is based on a person's age as indicated in Table 12.3.[412] To break this down, for adults between the ages of 18 and 59, the recommendation is 150 minutes a week of moderate physical activity, which is equivalent to 3 to 6 METs. But if someone performs vigorous physical activity for the cardioprotective benefit, 75 to 150 minutes is enough per week.

Other Added Benefits of Cardio

Rigorous data shows cardio not only improves our heart health, but also leads to better surgical outcomes, improved postoperative recovery, and a decreased need for hospitalizations.[413] In addition, multiple studies have demonstrated a clear correlation between regular physical activity and a reduced incidence of depression.[414]

Physical Activity and Depression

Every time we move our bodies, chemicals are released. Either the presence or absence of these chemicals impacts our brain. Our hypothalamic-pituitary-adrenal axis can be affected, helping us feel less stress and possibly lessening depression and anxiety.[408] Brain-derived neurotrophic factor (BDNF) is a growth factor in our brains associated with neuroplasticity (see Chapter 2: Lifestyle Psychiatry and Brain Health).[415] Exercise increases the level of BDNF as well as the release of endocannabinoids from the brain.[416] Exercise can also mitigate depressive symptoms by decreasing an inflammatory pathway in our skeletal muscles and increasing circulating cortisol in our brains.[417]

Though I mentioned earlier that light physical activity is not as protective as moderate and vigorous exercise, it's worth noting that even light activities, if done enough, can be cardioprotective.[418] The key is usually to be consistent.

Take the First Step—with Walking!

Walking can be an accessible and fun physical activity with potential benefits that should not be overlooked.

Historically, light physical activities have a lower dropout rate and less chance of injury. They also tend to be helpful for building relationships. I know so many people who have started taking phone calls or meetings while walking. Meeting others for a walk, instead of a lunch meeting, is another approach to nurturing social connectedness. What's important is keeping these ideas at the forefront in our day-to-day lives and using them to guide our choices.

Table 12.3 Physical Activity Guidelines Based on Age[412]

Age	Guidelines
Preschool-aged children (ages 3-5)	Preschool children should be physically active throughout the day and encouraged to participate in active play.
Children and adolescents (ages 6- 17)	Children and adolescents should include the following: Cardio: At least 60 minutes of physical activity each day. Most activity should be moderate or vigorous cardio activity, with vigorous physical activity at least 3 days each week. Muscle-strengthening: Muscle-strengthening physical activity at least 3 days each week. Bone-strengthening: Bone-strengthening physical activity at least 3 days each week.
Adults	Adults should move more and sit less throughout the day, with the following: Cardio: At least 150-300 minutes of moderate-intensity OR 75-150 minutes of vigorous-intensity cardio each week (or an equivalent combination). Muscle-strengthening: Activities of moderate or greater intensity involving all major muscle groups at least 2 days a week.
Older adults	If older adults are able to sustain moderate or vigorous exercise, they should incorporate multi-component physical activity (involving balance training) with the following: Cardio: At least 150-300 minutes of moderate-intensity OR 75-150 minutes of vigorous-intensity cardio each week (or an equivalent combination). Muscle-strengthening: Activities of moderate or greater intensity involving all major muscle groups at least 2 days a week. Importantly, older adults should determine their level of effort for physical activity and movement relative to their fitness level.
Women during pregnancy and the postpartum period	Women during pregnancy and the postpartum period should incorporate the following: Cardio: At least 150 minutes of moderate-intensity cardio activity each week. If women were engaged in vigorous-intensity cardio activity prior to pregnancy, they can continue these exercises during pregnancy as tolerated.

Table 12.3 Physical Activity Guidelines Based on Age (continued)	
	Women who are pregnant should consult their healthcare provider to determine if they should adjust their physical activity during pregnancy.
Adults with chronic health conditions or physical limitations	If adults with chronic conditions or physical limitations are able to sustain moderate or vigorous exercise, they should incorporate the following: **Cardio:** At least 150-300 minutes of moderate-intensity OR 75-150 minutes of vigorous-intensity Cardio each week (or an equivalent combination) **Muscle-strengthening:** Activities of moderate or greater intensity involving all major muscle groups at least 2 days a week. Importantly, when adults with chronic conditions or physical limitations are unable to meet the above guidelines, they should engage in regular physical activity and movement according to their abilities and conditions.

Table 12.3 adapted from U.S. Department of Health and Human Services, "Physical Activity Guidelines for Americans, 2nd edition," 2018, page 8-9

At some point in my life when I decided to change my couch potato ways, I started my walking program slowly, using the "rule of 2 and 3 miles per hour."[419] This rule is the recommendation for those of us who are suffering with cardiac issues or those who may be unfit, older adults, overweight, or obese. When we're walking outside, we should walk on level ground. Over time, we can increase the slope (grade) to an incline, but only if it feels manageable and is approved by our healthcare providers. There is a big jump in METs for every 1% change in the incline's grade, so it's important to start with a level grade and progress slowly, keeping to what's comfortable.[420] For example, if someone is walking at 2.5 miles per hour at a 1% grade, that's the equivalent of 2 METs. At a 4% grade, that's 4 METs. Though these changes in the level grade from 1% to 4% appear small, the METs moved from light to moderate!

I know I said this before, but it's worth repeating. The best rule of thumb when starting exercise is to first get cleared by our health providers. Once we're physically cleared, always start slowly.

We know we're engaging in light exercise if we can still talk and sing without being short of breath. Moderate exercise is if we can talk, but not sing while exercising. During vigorous exercise, it's difficult to both talk and sing.

Another important aspect to consider during physical activity is our maximal heart rate, which varies based on age. The American Heart Association has developed guidelines for target heart rates during exercise, which are displayed in Table 12.4.[421] According to the guidelines, for a 70-year-old, a heart rate above 150 bpm is never recommended, whereas for those between 20 to 40 years old, that is within the target range for cardio. However, if you have a heart condition or a medical condition, or if you take medications that affect your heart rate, this does not apply. Please discuss the target and maximum heart rates with your physician.

HIIT

Are you up for a challenge?

HIIT, which stands for High-Intensity Interval Training, is currently a popular training style for physical activity.[422] In HIIT, bouts of moderate activity—during which we are operating at 50 to 85% of our maximal heart rates, per Table 12.4—are separated by rest periods.

Research studies have highlighted the benefits of HIIT, showing that we can achieve comparable results in a shorter duration of time than needed with straight continuous training to achieve the same results.[423,424] An added benefit of HIIT is the reported increase in post-exercise oxygen consumption, which could potentially promote further weight loss.[425]

The biggest downside of HIIT is that it isn't recommended—and could even be dangerous—for patients with any heart disease, or those with inadequate cardiac conditioning who do not monitor their heart rate carefully.[437] Given this disclaimer, and with careful monitoring, many of my patients have found HIIT well-suited for their needs. In fact, for those of us for whom time constraints legitimately impact our ability to exercise, sneaking in 10-minute bursts of HIIT two or three times a day is a solid option.

Table 12.4. Target and Maximum Heart Rates by Age During Exercise in Beats Per Minute (bpm)[421]		
Age	Target Heart Rate Zone 50-85%	Maximum Heart Rate 100%
20 years	100-170 bpm	200 bpm
30 years	95-162 bpm	190 bpm
35 years	93-157 bpm	185 bpm
40 years	90-153 bpm	180 bpm
45 years	88-149 bpm	175 bpm
50 years	85-145 bpm	170 bpm
55 years	83-140 bpm	165 bpm
60 years	80-136 bpm	160 bpm
65 years	78-132 bpm	155 bpm
70 years	75-128 bpm	150 bpm

Table 12.4 adapted from American Heart Association, "Target Heart Rates Chart."

2. Strength Training

The goal of strength training is not to look like a bodybuilder—unless you want to!

Strength training has been historically controversial as an approach to overall health. Many people have looked down upon it as "just about appearance," rather than a crucial method for achieving optimal health. However, the benefits of strength training vary depending on age.

Strength Training: Older Adults

How much strength training do we need? As we age, we lose muscle, and therefore strength training is absolutely recommended for middle age and beyond. Low weights with multiple repetitions twice to three times a week are recommended for preserving our muscle mass and bone health. Consistently engaging in this practice as we age can enhance mobility and overall balance, resulting in fewer falls.[427]

Strength Training: Active Adults

Many personal trainers strongly advocate for building muscle, which can be helpful for younger people in burning off calories and stabilizing weight. But clearly, strength training doesn't offer the same benefits for heart health as aerobic training. I've met many personal trainers and fitness fanatics who engage in strength training five days a week but can't walk five miles at a vigorous pace because they haven't trained their hearts. Similarly, solely focusing on aerobic activity could lead to losing muscle strength as we age. Therefore, the American Heart Association recommends incorporating strength training into our weekly regimen about twice a week.[428]

3. Flexibility

How many people over the age of 50 can touch their toes? Not many. Why is this a problem?

Flexibility is the third component of physical activity. It's important for many reasons, including helping with joint health to avoid the risk of injuries and enhance the range of motion of our joints and muscles. This becomes especially important in a sedentary world, where we often sit in front of computers all day long and, over time, become predisposed to poor posture and chronic pain.

Some interesting research indicates that flexibility plays a substantial role in improving physical performance with higher levels of endurance and power.[429] For example, Olympic athletes and professional ball players all incorporate flexibility training into their weekly regimen.

For our heart health, flexibility is extremely helpful in enhancing circulation and oxygen delivery to muscles, and therefore helps the overall function and recovery of our body.[430] On the mental health side, research shows that flexibility reduces tension headaches and chronic pain conditions by promoting relaxation and mitigating stress. As we age, just as with strength training, flexibility becomes even more vital for maintaining an independent lifestyle.[431] Some highly recommended activities to improve flexibility include general stretching, yoga, and Pilates.

4. Balance

Balance is the ability to maintain stability while we are still or moving. Balance activities are extremely important for older adults and children, and they can decrease the risk of falls and associated injuries.[432] Many balance-strengthening movements are integrated into commonly performed physical activities. For example, ballroom dancing combines cardio and balance training. Yoga and tai chi often incorporate the act of standing on one leg to enhance balance. Balance training can be static (where we're not moving when we do the exercise) or dynamic (where we're moving or walking).

5. Speed

The speed of our movement is a vital component of physical activity.[433] For some of us who may have health conditions, our speed should be maintained at a manageable level. For those of us who have no significant health limitations, after starting slowly, increasing our speed can be another parameter we track.[434] For example, walking with an initial speed of 2 miles an hour can be incrementally increased as part of goal-setting to include a goal that is challenging yet attainable.

Final Thoughts

Many assessments are publicly available to evaluate our current state of physical activity and develop a plan to move forward. While tracking our health is a popular thing to do, please beware that tracking your weight, for example, is not the same as setting a goal. Goals should be based on things you do, not about the number on a scale. And, the ultimate goal in cardio is not weight loss but rather to improve cardiac function.

One of the most important parts of changing behavior is making sure that the goals are challenging but attainable as described in Rx 9.4. Wearable devices such as pedometers, fitness watches, etc., can hold us accountable while also providing a fun way to share progress with family and friends. In some European countries, there are entire community-based interventions incentivizing physical activity in enjoyable and engaging ways. For instance, machines in train stations in India offer free tickets if someone does 30 squats in 3 minutes, and accessible bikes have become part of the culture of the Netherlands. Even in the United States, many parks have incorporated small, accessible areas with exercise machines.

In this chapter, we have discussed many aspects of physical activity and goal setting so that you are empowered with the information. Hopefully, you are inspired to make changes to your routine or to continue your journey in physical activity. To put it all together, Rx 12.1 provides practical strategies that may help you achieve these goals.

R_X 12.1 Practical Strategies to Increase Your Physical Activity
Prescription

- Identify your "Why?" Refer to Rx 9.2.
- Create a list of physical activities you enjoy.
- Use Rx 12.2 to assess if you're ready to make a change.
- Start by incorporating a physical activity you enjoy doing.
- Set your goal using Rx 9.4.
- If you have injuries or physical limitations, please start small and go slowly.
- Once it feels right, find an activity partner, family member, or group that you can join. We will discuss this further in Chapter: 14 Connectedness.
- Give yourself positive affirmations and healthy feedback for progress.
- Consider charting your progress or recording your achievements.
- If you hit a plateau, consult a friend or expert for ideas. You could also try changing your activity and/or goals.
- As always, make sure to involve your healthcare provider who can monitor you with periodic testing, such as blood pressure, blood sugar, cholesterol, and fitness.

Chapter 13: Stress Management

Stress is like air—it's everywhere.

Stress is the most common symptom causing problems in the patients I see, and it likely affects a significant portion of the population, many of whom never make it to a psychiatrist's office. One of the major challenges with stress is that it gets in the way of us performing the tasks that may help us regulate our stress. When we're under stress, it can be difficult to handle even one extra item on our to-do lists. This is why we have talked about stress in other chapters when we discussed mental blocks.

Overview of Stress

Stress is our body's response to life changes or pressure.

Stress is a term used a lot in academic papers and in popular publications, and I want to clarify the science behind it in this chapter. I will discuss other terms used in the scientific literature too, including wellness, well-being, coping, and resiliency. Once we've defined some of these terms, we'll move on to discuss how each of us can identify where we are on the spectrum from "needs improvement" to "better" to "best" health, and from "less healthy" to "healthy" to "healthiest" coping strategies. Then we can begin developing and implementing healthy responses to stress.

How We Experience Stress

Overall, we can experience stress in multiple ways, including brief and transient stress, recurrent episodic stress, and lingering chronic stress:[435,436]

- *Acute stress* involves our sympathetic nervous system in response to immediate stressors, such as getting a tooth pulled or cutting ourselves. Our bodies do respond, though only briefly.

- *Episodic stress*, as the name implies, happens acutely but recurs over a series of episodes. This could be a pattern in our lives like dealing with traffic, which can repeatedly trigger a stress response. Or a newborn baby crying for two hours every day and the mother can't figure out what's wrong.
- The third major type of stress is called *chronic stress*. In this type, the initial cause is gone, but we're still experiencing the stress. Just remembering the event can even trigger a stress response. This can happen after individual traumatic experiences. But we can also observe this after larger events, like the COVID-19 pandemic. Burnout, which was described in Chapter 7, is related to chronic stress, but as mentioned before, the term is used in the medical literature to describe chronic stress originating from work-related situations.

Good versus Bad Stress

In her book G*ood Anxiety: Harnessing the Power of the Most Misunderstood Emotion*, Wendy Suzuki says, "When we have just the right kind or amount of stress in our lives, we feel balanced—this is the quality of well-being we always seek."[437]

In 1967, Holmes and Rahe developed a scale based on the concept that eustress ("good stress") and distress ("bad stress") are both factors affecting our lives.[438] The Holmes-Rahe Scale is a 43-item self-assessment of one's life stress. This scale asks us to identify both positive and negative life events during the past year, and a number value is assigned to each event. Examples of life events are marriage, divorce, pregnancy, outstanding personal achievement, changing one's line of work, etc. Though some of these life events are positive and some are negative, they are all considered stressful.

On the Holmes-Rahe Scale, a score of 150 points or less indicates a low chance of stress-induced health breakdown in the next two years. A score of 150 to 300 is associated with a 50% chance of health breakdown in the next two years. A score of 300 or more suggests an 80% chance of health breakdown in the next two years. Please note, this scale has been revised over the years by multiple authors in order to modernize it.[439,440] In the forthcoming story, I used the original scale since it was freely available at the time.

My 2023 Stress State

Psychiatrist, heal thyself.

In October 2023, as I was sitting down to review a draft of this chapter, curiosity led me to take the Holmes-Rahe test for myself again. It had been a while since I had taken the test. In my 20s and 30s, my score was through the roof—300 or so. However, recently, it seemed like my stress was minimal because I was in a more stable place, both professionally and personally. Yet, in 2023, I experienced a series of unrelated events that I didn't have time to fully process because I was juggling finishing two academic books and writing this book, in addition to my day job and other professional and personal commitments.

To my own surprise, shock, and embarrassment, my Holmes-Rahe turned out to be over 680. Wait, *what*? I have *at least* an 80% chance of a health breakdown in the next two years? I reflected on this and did an inventory of how I was doing. While I was functioning at work and actively engaged in drafting this book, there were multiple areas in my life over the previous few months that should've given me reason to pause. I was more direct than normal (I am a New Yorker, after all!) and abrupt with a few of my colleagues in meetings, so much so that I felt the need to apologize to them after the fact. I also found myself falling back into my old bad habits of not taking care of myself and skipping the gym.

After about four or five years of not having a cold, I developed an upper respiratory infection that just wouldn't go away and ultimately needed steroids and an inhaler.

What was my Rx? I realized I needed to declutter my work life and get rid of things I absolutely didn't have to do, so I could give my body time to heal, both physically and mentally. Although the stressors were real, I was so caught up in getting work done that I was disregarding the impact on my physical and mental health. Throughout my life, it had always been easier for me to work harder during times of stress. However, I realized that gave me little room to reflect and take the pause with intention I so desperately needed. Many of us continue to function, even with all these stressors in our lives, but then are surprised when our bodies break down.

Maybe we all need to hear this: Please heal thyself!

Wellness

Wellness is defined as a state of positive health characterized by a good quality of life and a sense of well-being. Wellness goes beyond simply an absence of disease or suffering—it's a dynamic state of being human that includes our relationship with the outside world. Given the complexity of our multiple relationships—personal, work, and community, as will be defined in Chapter 14: Connectedness—wellness can be difficult to research.

How does one devise a study investigating all the social aspects of a person's life? That's why we say wellness is somewhat of a *fuzzy concept* in research. Thus, researchers tend to use a different term that is easier to describe: *well-being*. The American Psychological Association describes well-being as a state of contentment and happiness, a good quality of life, a positive outlook, stable mental and physical health, and minimal distress.[441]

Stress, of course, is a common factor affecting our well-being, and is defined as a reaction to internal or external stimuli. What happens in our bodies to produce such reactions when we experience stress?

Our Body's Response to Stress

The current siloed diagnostic criteria for the cause of diseases may be too simplistic.

Our body has many ways of responding to stress, including palpitations, sweating, and dry mouth. If this stress becomes severe, this can even progress to shock, with a physical decrease in blood pressure and body temperature, where our ability to regulate our states breaks down.[442] After some time, when our physical ways of coping with stress don't work, we quickly become exhausted. Mental responses to stress may include difficulty concentrating, mood changes, irritability, and poor sleep.

Previously we defined stress as acute, episodic, and chronic. A *stressor* is an external stimulus that triggers a stress *response* in a person, which is composed of their behavioral and physiologic reactions to the stressful situation.[443] An individual's reaction to stressful events is variable, meaning that the way we experience stress tends to look different from person to person. There are numerous factors that dictate what we feel when we are stressed, including personal influences such as genetics and the current level of burden or workload in our lives. On a larger scale, we can also be affected by our cultural environment and things like socio-economic status. For more information see Chapter 8.[444,445]

Stress is an adaptive process, one that evolved to help humans respond to threats in our immediate environment, giving us a sense of urgency and helping us to survive. And while stress can be adaptive short-term, chronic or excessive stress can be harmful and lead to various health issues, including cardiovascular disease, depression/anxiety, and weakened immune response.[446] Ultimately it is a question of balance—the context of the stress determines whether or not the stress response is a healthy response to a situation or something that may be more harmful long-term.

The Science of Stress

Persistent or recurring exposure to stress, leading to longer-lasting stress response called chronic stress, is seen as a result of repeatedly activating stress response pathways. Beyond that, certain stressors represent a threat to our sense of selves, such as our self-esteem or social status and these are known to factor heavily into the body's metabolic processes, including producing higher levels of cortisol and other hormonal changes[444,447,448] (discussed in Chapter 5). Excessive cortisol can lead to potential health issues, which over time can lead to insulin resistance in the body, a risk factor for chronic diseases such as Type 2 diabetes.[449]

When someone experiences daily or chronic stress in the workplace, not only can they experience burnout, as discussed in Chapter 7, but potentially lasting health and behavioral effects. In some cases, the overlap in what happens between our mental and physical bodies becomes blurred, and it can be hard to tell if our physical illnesses are originally from a physical or mental cause. Indeed, physical and mental illnesses are bidirectional.

As we've mentioned time and time again, our overall health includes both mental and physical health. It's never one or the other—it's always both! The good news is that current research in this area has demonstrated the connection to our bodies. We are coming to understand how cellular and molecular responses to stress affect our physical and mental health, due to the same underlying causes.[445,447]

Stress Eating

One of the most common coping mechanisms in reaction to stress is eating, usually referred to as *stress eating* (as well as *stress-induced eating, comfort eating,* or *emotional eating*). While this habit can function as short-term relief for a long-term problem, it often causes more issues than it fixes.

Eating sweet and fatty foods (or "comfort" foods) actually quickens feelings of psychological relief and minimizes the feelings brought on by stress, which is helpful short-term but can form long-term habits associating the consumption of ultra-processed foods with stress relief, ultimately creating more potential risks, including abdominal obesity and poor metabolic health. Stress has been found to increase consumption of unhealthy food and decrease consumption of healthy food, with individuals letting lifestyle goals slip in the face of the stressors in their lives.[450]

Already, we understand that prolonged exposure to stressors can have negative long-term consequences for our health. But habits formed to cope with these stressors can be similarly detrimental.

As we've discussed all throughout this book, I have struggled with stress eating, and it and my mood improved considerably when I removed ultra-processed food from my diet and exercised consistently.[451,452]

Grief

The death of a spouse is one of the most stressful events a person can experience, per research findings. The grief associated with this loss has been poorly understood, until recently. Studies have shed light on the connection between grief, depression, and inflammatory processes that can be detected in the blood.[453] For example, in 2019, Christopher P. Fagundes showed that, after the loss of a spouse, widows have an increased likelihood of heart problems and dying early. His research reveals that a specific pro-inflammatory cytokine in the blood, interleukin-6, or IL-6, is elevated in grieving spouses, with those higher on the grief scale having higher levels of this inflammatory marker.[453]

Caregiver Stress

Another manifestation of stress is caregiver stress. In the 21st century, many of us are struggling to manage our lives while taking care of our older loved ones. Globally, 10% of the population is over the age of 65, and this is expected to increase over the next few decades, especially in industrialized nations where the aging population is already 20%.[454] While advancements in medicine have helped people live longer, living longer comes with the need to have optimal health during those added years to maintain a good quality of life. As 95% of older adults over 65 are diagnosed with at least one chronic condition and 80% have two or more chronic conditions, caring for older adults may be stretching us thin.[455] The stress is especially significant for the so-called "sandwich generation," middle-aged adults from the age of 40 to 59 who are supporting young children and their older parents.[456] To decrease the stress for the sandwich generation, support for the caregiver can be in the form of financial and emotional support, helping to expand this generation's resources and coping mechanisms.

A Note on Traumatic Mental Stress

In this chapter, we haven't discussed the importance of trauma as being a source of stress. It has not been forgotten, but because trauma can lead to such significant blocks in actualizing our potential, it was addressed separately in Chapter 3 on trauma as a mental block.

Social and Situational Factors

Our life's narrative is within our power to revise and *Restack*.
Demographic, socioeconomic, or simply environmental factors also play into our stress, as we explored in Chapter 8: Our Environment and Health. Though many of these factors may be out of our control, we do have the ability to change our internal relationship with them. This may involve claiming back our control through advocacy work and changing our own patterns.

My Case of Social and Situational Factors

In my case, my blocks and patterns were related to the abuse I endured in my marriage beginning as a late adolescent until I was 24. This trauma continued to shape the subsequent decades of my life, as I fell into a pattern of relating to others by giving more than I received and helping without getting anything in return. It differed from *altruism,* which is when you are primarily concerned of the well-being of others, especially people you don't know or expect to ever receive anything back from. In my case, I desperately wanted to connect with others in my life in a mutually loving way, therefore, I did want something in return for my kindness. Psychologically, this pattern served as an unconscious way for me to rewrite the narrative of my life and use my position of power and influence to right the wrongs done to me. Though I can never change my past and the things that happened, changing my future narrative *was* and *is* within my power. This can help make the past hold less weight in my life and be less triggering.

I share a few of the facts of my abuse to highlight the power of stress and trauma on our lives, even after the offending incident has passed. So much stigma surrounds people who have experienced abuse. Sometimes, the popular narrative becomes one of "once you've been abused, you abuse others." In my clinical practice, as well as in my personal life, I've seen the opposite more times than not. Indeed, changing our future narratives *is* within our power. As we revise and *Restack* ourselves, we can change the hold that the trauma and the traumatic patterns of repetition compulsion have on us and stop it from being passed on to future generations.

Resilience

We can't always control our circumstances, but we can become more *resilient*. Resilience describes the way we adapt—both within ourselves and in our external actions—to stressful experiences. The more resilient we are, the more flexible we are.

When I work with patients to help them cope and improve their mindset, resilience is what we're trying to cultivate—to increase their flexibility and approach to the situation. Often, we can't change our lives. Our environment and its stressors are already there, and we can only manage, at least initially, how we respond.

Coping as a Way of Building Resilience

Choose well! The effects of the coping strategies we adopt now can have long-lasting effects on our well-being, even decades later.

Many of us enter adulthood with firmly set ways of dealing with life's stresses. We often don't spend too much time reflecting on our coping. Still, taking a moment to identify what strategies we're using could go a long way in establishing novel approaches to deal with stressful situations in a healthier manner.

Coping is a well-studied concept. We described coping in Chapter 4: Emotion Regulation. Here, we'll expand on this concept and emphasize its role in building resilience. Overall, coping can be categorized by healthy or unhealthy practices we implement.[457]

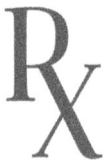

R℞ 13.1 Practicing Positive Cognitive Restructuring

Prescription

1. Bring a stressful situation to mind, or bring your awareness to the stress you feel in your day-to-day.
2. Normalize the experience of stress – everyone feels stress, and we all have it in our lives.
3. Acknowledge we're not perfect, and our lives are not perfect.
4. Consider that perfectionism may be a goal causing you undue stress.
5. Reframe your perspective by reminding yourself that being perfect is unattainable.
6. Make an active effort to work toward personal happiness each day of your life.
7. Identify and focus on aspects of your life that are under your control.

The six types of coping are:[458,459]

- *Positive cognitive restructuring* (working hard to focus on the positive and approach every situation with optimism), which involves the shifts in our mindset as we describe in Rx 13.1
- *Problem-solving* (strategizing, planning, seeking to resolve the underlying stressor)
- *Seeking support* (from family, peers, God, seeking advice and comfort from others)
- *Distraction* (when all else fails, sometimes it's easier to cope by engaging in healthy pleasurable activities like hobbies, TV, social media, and reading)
- *Escape/avoidance* (an effort to disengage cognitively or stay away; this may include denial and wishful thinking)
- *Self-blame and blaming or arguing with others* (deflecting the real issue or the resulting emotions)

Escape and avoidance are not as healthy in most situations. If we find that our coping mechanisms are not working, it may be because we are using less healthy coping strategies like escape and avoidance. When we observe this, it can be useful to try to implement more of the "healthiest coping strategies" as listed in Rx 13.2.[460]

R̶X 13.2 Reflecting on Your Coping Strategies[460]
Prescription

1. The table below has three columns of coping strategies: Less healthy coping, healthy immediate-relief coping, and healthiest coping. Imagine scenarios in your day-to-day life and note how often you use the specific coping strategy on a scale from 1-5 (with 1 being no use and 5 being very frequent use).
2. Keep track of how many *less healthy* coping strategies you employ.
3. Reflect on instances where you can change your approach and adopt healthier coping strategies.

Less Healthy Coping Strategies	Healthy Immediate-Relief Coping Strategies	Healthiest Coping Strategies
Unhealthy substance use	Humor	Planning
Denial	Venting	Problem-solving
Avoidance	Receiving emotional support	Positive reframing/optimism
Behavioral disengagement	Reaching out for help	Acceptance
Self-blame	Religion, spirituality, or connection with a higher power	Religion, spirituality, or connection with a higher power
Blaming or arguing with others	Self-distraction	Healthy exercise or physical movement
Isolating	Restful sleep	Eating healthy foods
Overeating, overworking, over-spending, etc.	Changing the stressful external environment	Participating in a hobby or sports

A Case of Replacing Coping Strategies

Miranda is a 38-year-old administrator with two small children who was going through a separation and subsequent divorce. She was raised in a close-knit family in Colorado. Two months ago, she found out her grandmother was developing Alzheimer's. Then, a week later, her beloved Uncle Billy died in a car accident. She was given a promotion at work two weeks ago and was praised at that time for her excellent work-life balance.

Miranda's truth was that she found herself *drinking* every night after the kids went to bed. She came to me for psychiatric help in tears, saying, "Nobody knows what I really feel." She said she was feeling overwhelmed with her responsibilities, including her volunteering position at the food bank. She used to find such joy with the shifts in the food bank and usually never said no in the past, but was overwhelmed as they asked her to take on more shifts. Volunteering was now starting to feel like a burden.

During our conversation, we worked to identify her coping strategies, and Miranda realized how much she was utilizing *avoidance* and *denial* in her current challenging emotional state. While she was receiving validation at her job and through volunteering, she was neglecting her hurt and pain about her divorce, her grandmother's dementia, and her uncle's death. She *blamed herself* for not being a good enough parent, since she was so busy all the time. Miranda also wasn't comfortable reaching out to her family members to tell them about her pending divorce. Through our conversations, she realized she needed to put her volunteering commitments on hold so she could prioritize her well-being and her family.

Miranda slowly got more comfortable using her *social network for support,* attending *religious services* with her kids every Sunday, where she began *developing a community* with fellow parents. She carved out time to *laugh and play* with her kids every day, and they began learning to *cook healthy meals* together. Miranda began to *accept her reality with the pending divorce* and started to *plan* for her future. Sometimes, she would come to the sessions with a newfound enthusiasm in her voice, exuding optimism as she spoke about her life.

After reading the case of Miranda, use Rx 13.2 to reflect on your current coping strategies. Consider healthier approaches you can adopt in response to stress in your life.

Rx 13.3 Reflecting on Your Mindset
Prescription

1. Call to your attention an event that happened recently that was bothersome. This is known as the activating event.
2. Identify your unwanted emotions during the event.
3. Note the beliefs you have surrounding the event. These are known as automatic thoughts.
4. Assess your behavioral and emotional responses by asking yourself the following:
    a. Are my responses irrational?
    b. Is there a way to modify how I'm thinking and feeling?
    c. Can I change the consequence in my mind through a more positive reframe, even though I may not be able to change the external environment? For example, "I'm annoyed that I have to drive my family member to an appointment every week" can be reframed to "I'm so fortunate to have a family whom I love and I can help."
    d. Is there a way to actually change my environment to minimize the activating event?
5. Identify other potential explanations for the scenario.
6. Make a list of all the possible other explanations that are more positive.
7. Consider responses that are more embedded in kindness and compassion for yourself.

An Approach to Shift Your Mindset

Reflection and *Restack*-ing is a path to un-set a set mind. Our mindset is key when we try to make changes. To shift our mindset, we need to consider multiple aspects of an approach initially developed by Albert Ellis and Martin Seligman.[461,462] This approach was further refined in a book by Carol Dweck called *The Growth Mindset*.[463] By using Rx 13.3, we can identify our emotions and beliefs and evaluate our responses with the goal of enhancing our mindset.

A Case of Reflecting on Our Mindset

Lucas is a 47-year-old nurse who describes himself becoming angry when a patient's family eats in front of a patient who is not allowed to eat before surgery. Lucas's beliefs include that the family is being inconsiderate, the family should eat elsewhere, it bothers the patient, and the patient might be tempted to break their fasting state. We usually call these beliefs "automatic thoughts." The consequences are that Lucas becomes annoyed with the patient's family, rolls his eyes upon entering the patient's room, and slams the door as he leaves. As Lucas worked through and reflected on his behavior and mindset, he was able to identify alternative scenarios that could be a more positive way to view the situation. For example:

1. Eating together is an important part of the patient's social connections.
2. The family was trying to be loving and normalize the evening ritual with the patient.
3. The patient asked the family to bring home-cooked meals, without realizing it wasn't allowed before surgery.
4. The family suffers from housing insecurity and doesn't have another safe place to eat.

Lucas was able to see that many other positive possibilities existed too. By using techniques like those outlined in Rx 13.3, Lucas gained insight into his automatic thoughts and recognized that some of his beliefs might be irrational or influenced by bias. He then began the process of improving his emotional response and practicing more kindness and empathy toward his patients' families. What a lovely *Restack*.

Examples of Coping Strategies

In Rx 13.1, we practiced positive cognitive restructuring. Most of us have heard of some of the coping strategies related to this concept of positive cognitive restructuring, such as gratitude, meditation, and mindfulness. We may have even tried them at some point. But these terms are so commonly used in everyday conversation that their importance and their potential impact on changes in brain structure are often lost.

Gratitude

Gratitude involves reframing our struggles and adopting a life orientation focused on the positives in the world. Over time, practicing gratitude can lead us to experience more social support and well-being. Rx 13.4 provides suggestions for ways to practice gratitude.

Meditation

Functional magnetic resonance imaging (fMRI) of the brain reveals that meditation activates parts of our brain involved in attention and arousal, and can therefore quiet our stress response.[464,465] Once activated by meditation, these brain regions—particularly the frontal, parietal, and cingulate cortex—can lower heart rate, improve blood pressure, and alleviate many physical symptoms of stress.[466] With consistent meditation practice, permanent structural changes in these regions of the brain regions can occur over time. Indeed, many long-term meditators are noted to have a thicker cortex, indicating sustained changes that can be attributed to a persistent, disciplined state of calmness.[466,467]

R̷ **13.4 Ways to Practice Gratitude**
Prescription

---

1. Make a vow or a **commitment** to practice more gratitude in your life.
2. **Write down** three things you're grateful for every morning.
3. **Add an appointment or reminder** on your calendar (weekly or monthly) to send an email or text to a colleague or friend, expressing gratitude to them. Be as specific and positive as possible.
4. **Express gratitude** to strangers or people you don't normally thank. For example, the cashier at the grocery store, the mailman, your parents or children.
5. **Practice a gratitude meditation.** Find a quiet spot and bring to mind things you are grateful for.
6. **Experience** the joy when others show gratitude to you. Breathe in, allow yourself to feel the positive feelings, let others know how their gratitude makes you feel, and express gratitude back if you are able.

Meditation Is *Not* a Religious Practice

One of the biggest hurdles to meditation that I've noted in my patients is the misconception that it's inherently tied to spirituality or religion. While much of mindfulness and meditation originated from Eastern religious traditions, they can be practiced in a secular manner as well. Research has demonstrated some positive effects of meditation for well-being.[468] It's important to separate this tool from religious practice in our minds so we can reap its benefits. Although mastering meditation requires regular practice—just like any other skill like riding a bike or training for a marathon—the benefits are enormous, even with just a few minutes a day of practice.

There are many ways to practice meditation. Most importantly, if one approach doesn't work for you, consider trying another. Rx 13.5 describes one specific method of practicing meditation—through focusing on our breathing.

℞ 13.5 Practicing Meditation
Prescription

1. Find yourself a comfortable place to sit, lie down, or stand.
2. Put on some calming music if you find that helpful.
3. Turn your attention to your breathing. Observe your breathing without changing anything.
4. Notice how the breathing feels in your body. It's important to focus on the sensations.
5. If your mind wanders, just notice that and bring your attention back to your breath.
6. Practice kindness with yourself as you continuously bring yourself back to your breath.

Mindfulness

Mindfulness is different from meditation in that it involves awareness of our thoughts, emotions, and experiences. However, mindfulness and meditation may share similar strategies, such as mindfulness meditation, which is exploring patterns of thinking and body awareness.

John Kabat-Zinn developed mindfulness, distilling it into an easy-to-follow, eight-week protocol called mindfulness-based stress reduction (MBSR), which has been shown to lead to lasting improvements in well-being by altering brain structure.[469,470] Similar to meditation, MBSR has been noted to cause changes in the gray matter of the brain and enhances emotion regulation, memory, and learning.[471] As a bonus, MBSR also fosters our self-compassion (discussed in Chapter

14: Connectedness), thereby promoting a growth mindset.[471] Though we can find MBSR groups online or in person, there are also free resources (such as www.palousemindfulness.com) so you can become an expert and share the techniques with others.[472]

Stress Is Complex

Stress has significant and potentially long-lasting effects on our body. It often takes months to years to build up to the bundle of stress that many of us become, yet we want a quick fix. The bad news is that only a few quick fixes are available. The good news is if we implement some of the techniques in this chapter, we can find ourselves de-stressing and ultimately able to better *Restack* ourselves. Of course, many of us may need professional help, which we will discuss in Chapter 16: Beyond Self-Help. I know for myself, my stress has been so interconnected with others in my life that to unwind its effects, I've had to deal with the concepts presented in the next chapter on connectedness.

Chapter 14: Connectedness

The population of the world continues to grow, yet individually, we are feeling more and more alone.

On May 1, 2023, the U.S. Surgeon General declared an epidemic of loneliness and isolation.[473] It may seem odd for loneliness to be considered a public health crisis since most of us are used to hearing about physical diseases as public health issues. However, as many of us (or someone we care for) have experienced, isolation can precipitate feelings of depression or anxiety.[474] If we are surprised by the framing of this public health crisis, it might be due to the common misconception that mental health disorders are separate from, and maybe less tangible than, our physical health. But connectedness (or the lack thereof) has a concrete impact on our overall health, both mental and physical.

While the U.S. Surgeon General's guidance is on loneliness and isolation, my bias is to broaden the focus to a term called *connectedness*. Connectedness encompasses not only social connection, but also our broader human connections including our relationship with ourselves. Given this framework, I believe the five aspects of connectedness are (1) social connection, (2) happiness, (3) empathy and compassion, (4) spirituality, and (5) purpose in life and meaning making. This is depicted in Figure 14.1.

So how does connectedness affect our health, and what interventions can we undertake to support our mental health through connectedness?

Social Connection Saves Lives

Loneliness is as dangerous as smoking 15 cigarettes a day.[475]

Social connection affects many areas of our life, including our body's biology, aspects of our psychology, and the way we relate to others behaviorally—all of these then affect our overall health and well-being. Social connection has been a hot area of research for decades.

COVID-19 brought to light some of the problems we face with social connection, in that many adults reported feeling a lack of connection with others and were experiencing low life satisfaction and heightened mental and physical health issues.

But these problems didn't start with COVID-19. The U.S. was already grappling with profound social isolation before the pandemic. A pre-pandemic survey, which investigated trends in social isolation between 2003 and 2020, revealed that we have been spending increasing amounts of time alone and less time in social engagements.[476] In more concrete terms, over those 17 years of the survey, our time spent alone increased by 24 more hours per month (15% increase), and social engagement with others decreased on average by 10 hours per month (20% decrease). This is especially alarming for young people ages 15 to 24, who spent 70% less time in person with friends in the years leading up to the pandemic.

Multiple studies have confirmed that a lack of social connection is as dangerous to the body as smoking up to 15 cigarettes a day or drinking six alcoholic drinks daily.[477] Lacking social connection is also more dangerous than physical inactivity, obesity, and air pollution, in terms of the odds of premature mortality. No wonder the U.S. Surgeon General is taking this problem so seriously and calling loneliness an epidemic!

The Impact of Social Connection on Overall Health

Have you ever noticed how much better you feel after spending an afternoon with good friends?

Why does our connectedness have such a significant impact on our overall health? To answer this, we have to examine three aspects of our overall health: psychological, biological, and behavioral aspects.

FIGURE 14.1 THE FIVE ASPECTS
OF CONNECTEDNESS

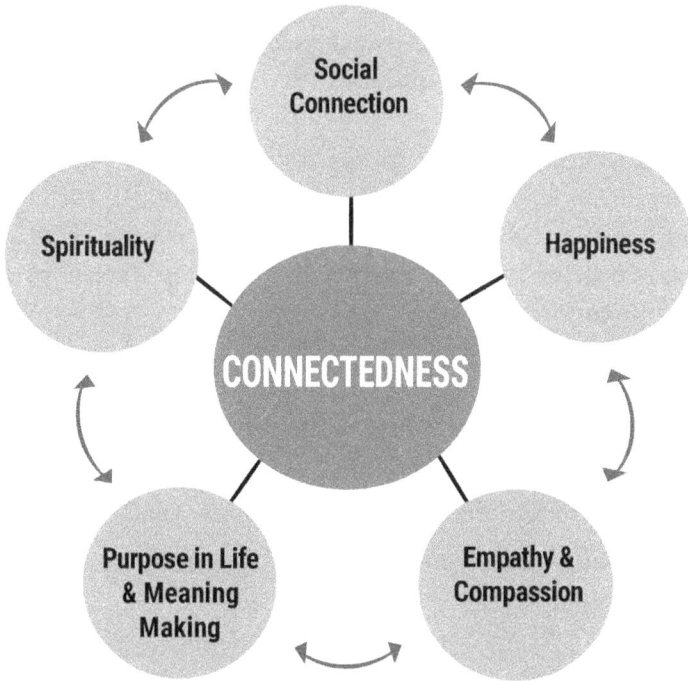

On a psychological level, our social connection influences our relationship to our life's meaning and purpose, resilience, hopefulness, experience of stress, and feelings of safety. Biologically, our stress hormones, inflammation, and gene expression are all affected by our social connections.[478] Lastly, social connection affects behaviors such as physical activity, nutrition, sleep, smoking, and the ability to receive treatment for mental health conditions.

When these aspects of our social connection are not in check, we become predisposed to serious health outcomes, such as heart disease, stroke, and diabetes, as well as overall premature death.[479] From a mental health standpoint, loneliness can have profound and pervasive consequences, including heightened levels of depression and anxiety, even among children.[480,481] One study involving 60,000 older adults demonstrated that increased loneliness was cited as one of the primary motivators for self-harm.[482]

Identifying the gaps we have in our connections is a valuable first step before we can seek solutions to what we're missing. Rx 14.1 prompts us to identify the size and quality of our social connections. This list will be useful as we delve into the chapter and develop a plan of action to enhance our connectedness.

As you work through Rx 14.1, pay close attention to any feelings associated with each connection you identify.

The Science of Social Connection

The threads of social connection weave themselves together and find their way into our brain.

Researchers are still trying to understand the changes social isolation creates in the brain. Some recent findings show that social connection is associated with an increased cortical thickness of the brain, which is important for our global thinking. Other changes noted include improved connectivity of regions of the brain and reduced symptoms of anxiety and depression in children.[483-485]

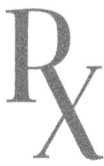

R℞ 14.1 Reflecting on Your Social Connections

Prescription

1. Consider the people you interact with regularly. Make a list.

2. Do you find the number of people to be to your liking, or would you like more or fewer?

3. Reflect on the quality of these relationships. Ask yourself if you're happy with them, or what you would change about them if you could.

4. Identify the following about your social network:

   a. Name of individual: List the people you would consider part of your social network. Include family, friends, colleagues, and mentors.

   b. Frequency of interaction: Some people we interact with daily, some people once a week, some people once a year, or maybe even less than that.

   c. The role they provide: People in our lives fill different roles. These roles can include those who provide us with emotional support, those we can rely on in a crisis, those who provide us with mentorship, those we can meet in person, those we can call anytime, or those who are more available virtually or through text.

   d. Quality of the relationship: Not all relationships are good for us. Consider if you feel happy and satisfied with the relationship, or if the relationship feels strained, difficult, one-sided, contentious, or abusive.

Studies have been able to connect social isolation with increased activation of the hypothalamus-pituitary-adrenal cortex (HPA) axis which is important in chronic stress.[486] While we need more research on this, this may indicate that social isolation has a functional and identifiable area in the brain we could target with treatment.

Early life stressors, such as exclusion or isolation from a social group, are known to produce many responses. We've discussed early life stress in terms of trauma in Chapter 3 and how it can lead to posttraumatic stress disorder and trauma reactions. But even early life stressors that don't rise to a formal trauma diagnosis can cause permanent changes in the immune function of the brain, affecting our HPA axis through elevated proinflammatory cytokines. This can ultimately contribute to vulnerability for developing heart disease, cancer, type 2 diabetes, fragility, age-related chronic diseases, and depression.[486]

The connection between social exclusion and inflammation was explored in a series of studies revealing that exclusion, or a lack of social connection, is linked to heightened inflammation, which could lead to depression.[487,488] Social exclusion was also found to be associated with increased fat stores, predisposing us to struggles with being overweight and obesity.[488]

Overall, the relationship between social isolation and inflammation in the body has been found to be bidirectional. On one hand, the emotional impact of isolation heightens inflammation. On the other hand, the physical symptoms of inflammation can intensify a person's isolation because the individual isn't feeling physically well enough to leave the home or engage with others. This can quickly become a vicious cycle.

Research Studies Using fMRI and Social Connection

We can now *see* the brain respond to connectedness.

With the advent of the fMRI scanner in the 1990s, the study of brain health became exponentially more exciting. Research in social connection and how it relates to our brain has arrived at a place where even the naysayers are beginning to believe. We have now reached a stage where much of the soft science of why relationships are important is finding a place in hard science.

One interesting study showed three children playing a game of Cyberball, a virtual ball-toss game.[489,490] Initially, all three children played together. But then, two of the children excluded the third from the game. The child who was rejected experienced emotional distress, as did the two children who were rejecting the third child. An fMRI scanner was used to track the children's brain responses. The emotional pain of being rejected activated the dorsal portion of the anterior cingulate cortex, which is the same brain region that perceives physical pain, rejection from a romantic partner, and bereavement and grief. The implications of this study are mind-boggling. If we're suffering from emotional pain, our experience of physical pain may be intensified, and vice versa—that is, if we're in physical pain, then our emotional pain feels more overwhelming. To the brain, rejection just plain hurts.

Reconsidering the Best Approach to Education

When many of us were growing up, socialization was not considered an important part of our education or our daily lives. In most countries, children are expected to sit still at a desk and complete assignments and tests individually. There is emerging research shedding light on the benefits of a different approach.

In 2022, a fMRI scan study of 50 children between the ages 8 to 12 assigned one group of students to complete a task with a peer, while the other group had to do it alone.[491] The students who worked with a peer enjoyed the task more and were able to complete it more quickly. These outcomes may suggest that learning with a peer may be superior and improve results in the classroom.

We often teach children to do things alone. But the question is, are these old paradigms losing their usefulness? Should we consider new ways of approaching education, taking the brain science on social connection more into consideration? In higher education, many instructors are revising their curriculum to include group learning, such as problem-based learning and small and large group discussions. Some instructors, who are aware of the science, have already been doing this for many years. As a potentially enjoyable practical exercise for our personal lives, try using Rx 14.2 as an opportunity to learn with someone.

R℞ 14.2 Learning Together
Prescription

---

1. Connect (via text, phone, email, video chat, etc.) with a friend or family member whom you enjoy spending time with (or lost touch with, or need an excuse to reconnect with).

2. Identify a topic or two that your friend or family member knows very well that you genuinely want to learn more about. Alternatively, suggest a topic both of you would like to learn more about.

3. Begin a conversation to learn more together, either via virtual meetings, phone calls, or in person. Email is usually less effective.

4. Set up regular times to talk, discuss, and do research together. Don't forget to make it fun! If possible, meet in nature or outside so you can both benefit from the synergy of nature and connectedness.

Happiness: The Science Behind It

Don't forget to connect with yourself, too.

While most authors would limit this chapter to just social connections, I believe the relationship we have with ourselves is a crucial aspect of connectedness.

Happiness, for instance, is primarily a relationship with ourselves, but can manifest as an aspect of socializing with others through our altruistic activities. Happiness is often described as a subjective state of well-being, and often related to our internal satisfaction with ourselves. It encompasses our values and is often based on an ability for us to manage our expectations as described below.

Happiness has been defined in a variety of ways throughout history and across cultures. According to Aristotle, happiness represents the highest aim of humanity and comprises two main components: *hedonia* (pleasure) and *eudaimonia* (a life well-lived). While pleasure in the day-to-day (hedonia) is still part of the conversation, a life well-lived (eudaimonia) is especially important to the state of happiness. A life well-lived is a philosophical concept emphasizing how vital it is to find meaning in our lives. Based on my experience, the most effective strategies for promoting the happiness of patients—the techniques that seem to have the greatest impact on brain structure—all relate to a larger sense of meaning. While happiness is described with connectedness, it is also related to our ability to cope and our sense of personal resilience. Resilience is a key for experiencing a sustained state of happiness–even in the face of adversity.

In Rx 14.3, you're encouraged to write your own obituary or eulogy.

R͟X 14.3 **Writing Your Own Obituary**
Prescription

After a long, happy, and fulfilling life and a joyous retirement, you pass away from natural causes. Reflect on your life in order to write your own obituary or eulogy. As you are completing this exercise, use the following questions to guide your thinking. Try not to overthink this and avoid critiquing your thoughts.

1. What would your life have been like?
2. What would you like to be remembered for?
3. What were some of your most challenging moments?
4. What was most meaningful for you in your life?
5. What gave you joy?
6. Whom did you impact in a positive way?

Did any aspect of this exercise surprise you? Responses typically vary from person to person. Still, your responses may help you pinpoint what truly matters to you. Did you mention family or friends? Were the imperfections that plague you now as important? Were the small, nit-picky fights you have with your loved ones even relevant?

Practically, How Do We Increase Happiness in Our Everyday Lives?

One surefire way to increase happiness—help someone!

Altruism is another strategy that can change our brains to increase our personal happiness. Multiple studies have found that altruistic emotions and behaviors not only make us feel better, but also contribute to longer and healthier lives. Altruism can cultivate positive emotions, which can then enhance our confidence, decision-making, and a sense of belonging and connectedness.

Some fMRI studies even show that if we engage in altruistic social activity, we end up having larger gray matter volume in certain regions of the brain associated with counteracting the effects of dementia.[492] Interestingly, the same benefits are not observed when we care for family or other people we know, where a relationship of mutual benefit exists. But individuals who performed altruistic things for people they didn't know, while receiving no reward, did improve the gray matter volume in certain regions of their brain, including the posterior insula, middle cingulate gyrus, hippocampus, thalamus, superior temporal gyrus, inferior orbital gyrus, and middle occipital gyrus.[492] Why am I mentioning all these regions of the brain in such detail? These brain regions have been brought up at multiple points in this book and are related to emotional trauma and cognitive illnesses like dementia. This is promising research because if altruism can be linked to these same regions of the brain, then we can potentially use this lifestyle strategy of altruism to improve our emotional traumas and cognitive illnesses.

In a similar study, it was noted that adolescents are extremely sensitive to altruism. On brain scans, altruistic activity lit up regions in the subjects' brains that aid in reward processing.[493] If we can encourage our adolescents to alter their mindsets and embrace altruistic behaviors, we're affecting—potentially permanently—their brains and brain health. This can help their brain grow and develop to be better prepared for making complex decisions later in life.

Laughter Therapy

Another intervention, even more concrete than altruism, is laughter therapy. How's laughter going to help us? It creates physical changes in our body and organs to reduce stress, increases endorphins in your brain, stimulates circulation, improves our immune function, and can improve feelings of sadness and anxiety. Fortunately, laughter therapy sessions are available worldwide, both online and in person. Try it out, you may get a good chuckle out of it.

Managing Expectations

Helping others and laughing increase our experience of happiness, but so can managing our expectations.

An important aspect of cultivating happiness is the concept of expectation management. A classic study of American adults between 1972 and 2004 showed that for every additional 10 years of life, the odds of being happy increased 5%.[494] The study found that older adults found greater contentment with their lives through adjusting their expectations. In practical terms, when we're younger and on the hedonic treadmill of career-building and chasing goals that are often out of reach, we tend to be less happy.

Rx 14.4 suggests ways to set more healthy expectations of yourself and others.

R℞ 14.4 Managing Your Expectations
Prescription

1. Either open your journal or find a quiet place to reflect.
2. Consider areas in your personal or professional life where you feel frustrated or dissatisfied.
3. Consider areas where you hold unrealistic expectations for yourself or others.
4. Reflect on your frustrations using Rx 3.1 Developing Your Double-Edged Sword Through the Reflect and *Restack* Cycle.
5. Ask yourself if the expectations are realistic, necessary, and/or important.
   a. If yes, connect with your feelings using Rx 4.1.
   b. If no, adjust your expectations by practicing more flexibility. After reflecting on Rx 14.3 Writing Your Own Obituary, imagine your life full of happiness, joy, and fulfillment.

Empathy and Compassion

Our humanness is elevated with every compassionate and empathic expression.

Broadly, empathy is the ability to imagine and understand the thoughts, perspectives, and emotions of another individual. However, fMRI studies have demonstrated multiple types of empathy—the research is ongoing, and in some studies, seven or more types of empathy have been identified! These different subcategories or types of empathy are encoded in different regions of the brain.[495] For example, *affective* empathy is the ability to feel another person's feelings. Mirror (or *motor*) empathy is the ability to replicate the behavior of another individual. *Mentalization* empathy is being able to infer someone else's behavior. *Cognitive* empathy is an understanding of others' feelings. What is clear is that someone might be stronger in one type of empathy but weaker in another.

Empathy and compassion are deeply intertwined since cognitive empathy is necessary before the response of compassion. Compassion is the actionable desire to help, either yourself or others, when moved by suffering or distress (in yourself or others). Therefore, empathy and compassion are essential aspects of how we relate to ourselves, through self-compassion and self-empathy, as well as those around us. Our ability to show empathy and compassion toward ourselves and others affects our capacity to develop meaningful connections. Compassion leads to positive feelings and protects us from burnout, as described in Chapter 7. Without a well-developed sense of compassion, our lives may feel shallow, and we may experience feelings of loneliness and isolation. With compassion, we increase our capacity for joy and love, contributing to a more fulfilling life.

Developing Empathy

Empathy is developed when we're toddlers. Some primitive forms of empathy are noted even a few hours after birth, as newborns respond more intensely to the sound of other babies crying compared to other noises. The latest research is just as clear: empathy can be taught, at least in a way that could change our compassion toward ourselves and others. There may be aspects in our lives where we feel blocked in our ability to be empathic with ourselves or others. Please rest assured that many of us can overcome this barrier through intentional training. In fact, at Harvard Medical School, thousands of clinicians are being trained by a course titled "Empathetics," which was developed by physician Helen Riess (www.empathetics.com).

Practical strategies to develop our empathy include:
1. Communication skills training
2. Watching theatrical performances
3. Exposure to positive role models
4. Reflecting on negative encounters with others
5. Practicing identifying facial expressions of others

6. Identifying non-verbal communication used by others
7. Studying literature and the arts
8. Recognizing our emotions and becoming more self-aware
9. Engaging in moderate or vigorous physical activity

We also know that people who engage in moderate or vigorous physical activity show significantly higher self-reported cognitive empathy when compared to people with low physical activity levels.[496] Indeed, physical activity not only aids in alleviating depression and anxiety, but also fosters social connection. Lifestyle interventions can influence empathy, therefore indirectly affecting connectedness.

A Note on Self-Compassion

Research shows that being compassionate with ourselves increases our endorphins and releases oxytocin, which helps our well-being and stops our fight-or-flight sympathetic response.[497] Self-compassionate people are better able to deal with stress and trauma and experience lower levels of anxiety and depression. For many people, especially those struggling with family obligations, it may feel selfish and unattainable to spend time taking care of yourself in this way. But understand that by practicing self-compassion, you're also helping your loved ones since you are emotionally healthier.

The structured resources for enhancing self-compassion require us to engage for a few minutes a day, but they can be tremendously helpful in various aspects of our lives. Kristin Neff and Christopher Germer are the gurus of self-compassion research and have developed a very valuable website, www.self-compassion.org.[498] This website is replete with free information including written and guided tools for the self-help practice of compassion.

Spirituality

Spirituality can be practiced through many seemingly unrelated activities, like riding a bike, running, meditating, or praying.

In this book, when we discuss spirituality, we're not strictly talking about religion, though religion may also be a type of spiritual practice. Religion is an organized belief system with rituals and connections to a higher power. In contrast, spirituality is a broader concept than religion. Spirituality encompasses multiple ways we express meaning and purpose, as well as connectedness to ourselves, others, nature, and *maybe* even a higher power. Embracing spirituality is crucial as it can improve lifestyle satisfaction and overall health, as well as manage depression and anxiety. Engaging in spiritual activity may impact the brain through brain-derived neurotrophic factor (BDNF), which is a hormone that plays a role in psychiatric disorders such as major depressive disorder, posttraumatic stress disorder, and substance use disorders.[499] We also know spirituality can help protect our heart health, though the effect of this may vary across different populations and cultures.

While many ordinary activities are not necessarily spiritual, for some people they can be if we practice them while being connected and ascribing meaning to them. Spiritual practices can span the gamut from running, walking, and yoga, to singing, chanting, meditation, mindfulness, prayer, and breathing exercises. I encourage readers to explore and engage in some activity they have a spiritual relationship with, whatever that may mean for them.

A Note on Nature as Medicine

A walk in the woods can be a most potent prescription.

It's become clear that there are numerous positive health benefits associated with spending time outdoors. *Forest bathing*, (known as Shinrin-yoku), rooted in Japanese traditions, is a way of calming ourselves and enhancing our sensory connection with nature.[500,501] In the

United States, this concept is also called forest therapy, where multiple organizations train guides to provide this experience. The Association of Nature and Forest Therapy (https://www.anft.earth/) report guides in 65 countries with numerous opportunities to find groups on their website. The practice involves an experience similar to meditation, wherein individuals take in the beauty of the forest and breathe in phytoncides, which are chemicals that plants emit to protect themselves from insects, but can be very beneficial to our immune system.[510,511] Many of the forest bathing groups walk and sit in silence, immersing themselves in the experience.

The basis of the healing property of nature is currently being studied by scientists. One study even noted that just removing our gaze from the computer and looking at a picture of nature for a few minutes a day has significant health benefits as well.[502] How does this happen? Researchers postulate that when our visual gaze is narrowed and focused, such as when working on a computer for hours a day, we deprive certain regions of the brain from receiving stimulation.[503,504] Looking away and expanding our visual field is part of the therapeutic benefit and helps reduce stress.

When looking at the benefits of being in nature, researchers turn to green spaces and blue spaces. Blue spaces refer to locations that are close to water, whether it is natural or man-made. Additionally, evidence shows those of us who live close to blue spaces engage in more physical activity and that the environment around these areas may be overall healthier.[505,506] Data also displays health benefits from being near green spaces, including improved activity in the amygdala, decreased cortisol levels, lower sympathetic activity and as mentioned earlier, an improved immune system.[507-509]

Our exposure to the healing benefits of phytoncides [510,511] also depends on the amount of time we spend in nature, with 120 minutes per week deemed as optimal.[512] For many of us, gardening is an accessible avenue for grounding ourselves in nature. Those who are located in urban areas won't have access to a forest, but they may have access to a community garden plot or planters. Additionally, there are numerous garden initiatives and urban garden programs implemented for socialization. Any gardener will share their experience with the therapeutic effects of working the soil with the hands—it's calming, rewarding, requires physical movement, and provides a direct connection with nature.[513] Of course, safety is an important consideration. Please keep in mind that being outdoors includes the risk of tick-borne illness, allergies, and other potential environmental hazards.

A Case of Bike Riding as a Spiritual Practice

Randi was a 23-year-old patient of mine who was initially very upset when I made a connection with their bike riding being a spiritual practice. They said, "That's not appropriate. I don't believe in God, and I'm not a spiritual being." But then we talked about how they loved to ride their bike every day. They would sometimes go on 5- or 10-mile bike rides and would "zone out" while connecting to nature. Randi reflected on the feelings of calmness, relaxation, and euphoria they experienced during these bike rides. We both grinned and agreed, Randi was indeed in a psychological space similar to what is experienced during prayer.

Spirituality in Adolescence

Spirituality can have a particularly pronounced benefit in adolescence because the brain is actively evolving during this time. Habits or thought processes adopted in adolescence can affect brain functioning for decades to come. These brain changes are noticed in the brainstem and basal ganglion and can aid adolescents in establishing and solidifying value-based goals for their lives.[514] This process often involves supportive relationships and engaging in deeper reflections about spiritual concepts. Spirituality thereby fosters connectedness on multiple levels in adolescents as they transition into adulthood.

Spirituality and Serious Illness

Medical institutions are beginning to recognize the importance of addressing the spiritual needs of patients. A recent study in JAMA looked at the connections between spirituality and serious illness and highlighted multiple glaring deficiencies, including the fact that many hospitals do not incorporate spiritual care while patients are hospitalized.[515] The data presented was clear—those who received spiritual care did better physically and mentally. While the hospital systems may not yet be ready to provide spiritual care for serious illnesses, we can provide this support for our loved ones. If you know someone who's struggling with their health, offering them resources to bolster their connection with a higher power or other forms of spiritual practices can be very therapeutic.

Purpose in Life and Meaning Making

Viktor Frankl, psychiatrist and Holocaust survivor, spoke about the centrality of meaning in his Holocaust experience. Meaning making gave him purpose in life, even in the most difficult of circumstances.
Meaning making refers to the process of how we understand and make sense of our life experiences and relationships. What we know from subsequent research is that creating meaning in our lives often leads to improvements in our well-being and feelings of depression and loneliness can decrease. How frequently we socialize also varies depending on whether we feel we have meaning in our lives.

Though the social and psychological impacts are compelling in and of themselves, having meaning in our lives also has a biological impact. For example, studies have linked meaning making with lower inflammation, as measured by a reduction of the inflammatory marker C-reactive protein, especially in older adults.[516]

So how do we develop meaning making? As I mentioned earlier, it involves engaging in activities that bring us fulfillment. This can be anything, for example, gardening, exercising, playing cards, dancing, playing an instrument, volunteering, teaching, or spending time with a pet. What do you consider meaningful and important to you?

Meaning Making at the End of Life

One study examined people with brain tumors who were not expected to survive more than five years.[517] Some of these patients had an existentially meaningful goal or activity to engage in. For some, it was gardening. For others, it was knitting or volunteer work. In each case, it was something the patient felt gave their life purpose and fulfillment. Patients who engaged in these kinds of activities not only improved their quality of life but also their survival time. Let's not minimize how important these interventions can be for us and our loved ones, especially in the case of terminal disease. Having a quality of life is a right until the end of life.

Conclusion

The domino effect of connectedness combats our epidemic of loneliness. Many aspects of connectedness involve a connection to ourselves and others. We also need to consider our connectedness to a higher power and spirituality. We cannot experience connection without having the traits of empathy and compassion. As we nurture our connectedness, it's important to manage our expectations, savor the moments of joy in our everyday lives, and seek purpose and meaning in our lives.

Ultimately, we all aim to live a fulfilling life. Stopping and pausing to reflect on how we envision the future narrative of our life through the obituary exercise in Rx 14.3 can allow us to watch this intention unfold. Hopefully, the science and data presented in this chapter will inspire you to change what you can. It's like a domino effect. Sometimes it just takes moving one domino to create a ripple effect of changes in multiple areas of our lives.

Chapter 15: Substance Use Harm Reduction

Love yourself enough to not harm your body with unhealthy substances. We have covered many different concepts in this book, and somehow, this is the hardest to write about. I find it so important, but this is the one chapter that tends to trigger many people. We don't want to get rid of the joy associated with drinking wine or beer, hanging out with our buddies at the bar, or taking shots with friends. These activities are associated with such happy times, until they're not so happy for some.

Substance use has overtaken much of society in an astounding manner. As a society, we struggle with the impact of the medical complications of substance use, car accidents while driving under the influence, the cost associated with lost days at work and doctor's appointments, and the devastating effects of uncontrolled behavior while intoxicated. Let's start first by exploring some of the data.

How Bad Is the Problem?

About 46 million individuals in the U.S. have a substance use disorder, of which about 30 million are related to alcohol, yet less than 10% receive any treatment.[518,519]

Alcohol use is associated with many chronic diseases that lead to a poor quality of life, including cirrhosis of the liver, heart disease, and cancer.[520] Overconsumption of alcohol is the leading cause of preventable disease in the U.S., with about 140,000 alcohol-attributed deaths per year, 1 out of 10 of which are fatalities resulting from traffic accidents.[521] Tobacco use is related to many of the same diseases as alcohol, and we can add tuberculosis and lung disease to that list.

While alcohol and tobacco use are heavily researched and receive considerable attention in the popular press, even more significant are the impacts of opioids (like heroin or fentanyl), prescription drugs, cocaine, and other misused substances. While this chapter does not aim to provide an exhaustive list of substances, and most of us are aware of the public health problems of substances, it feels incomplete without starting with some of their data.

It's beyond the scope of this chapter to write about the specific health consequences of substance use. Instead, I want to focus on exploring why substances can be so addictive and provide information for those who might be at risk of becoming addicted. I also want to give those who already struggle with unhealthy substance use, or those with family or loved ones with a substance use disorder, a starting point for thinking through their options.

The purpose of this discussion is not about judgment, but about mitigating harm. It's about *loving yourself enough to not want to harm your body.*

It's Not Your Fault

To be sure, there is plenty of research investigating the genetics underlying unhealthy substance use. Studies have identified multiple genes that can predispose people to substance use disorders. For example, in alcohol, the metabolizing genes ADH1B and ALDH2 are strongly associated with alcohol-use traits.[522] Having these genes does not necessarily mean someone will develop unhealthy use, but the struggle is more real for those with the genes.

A complex interplay occurs between our genes and the environment. While infants do not choose the family they're raised in, some data shows environmental exposure to caretakers who struggle with addictions can make the children more susceptible to unhealthy substance use.[523] This has been studied related to posttraumatic stress disorder and the concept of adverse childhood experiences (ACEs), particularly with children who are exposed to trauma in the home. The ACEs Questionnaire is an adult screening tool consisting of 10 categories of experiences. The higher a person scores on the ACEs, the higher the likelihood of having physical, mental, and substance use-related disorders. The website www.ACEsaware.org provides more information and resources about adverse childhood experiences and their potential consequences.

Some literature purports that epigenetic change, more specifically the environment in which a person was raised, is another important factor predisposing to substance use disorders.[524] *Epigenetics* refers to how our environment and our behavior can change the way our genes are expressed, without any changes to the genes themselves. Other commonly known epigenetic changes are autoimmune diseases and certain types of cancers.

Taking responsibility for our behaviors doesn't mean blaming ourselves. Many factors influence our unhealthy behaviors. But it is important to remain accountable for behaviors we can *Restack* as we continue on our journey of improving ourselves.

A "Little Substance Use"

We want to feel good, better, and happy. So, what's the harm?

Recreational substance use, though controversial, has become accepted by many in our society. I tend to agree there is no harm unless we're using substances that, for example, within several uses can activate areas of our brain involved in addiction and can therefore make us lose control of our behavior. Substance use can become an addiction in as little as a few uses or after years and addiction is defined as a chronic relapsing disorder. Addiction is characterized by compulsive substance seeking, continued use despite harmful consequences, and potentially long-lasting changes to the brain. By *Restack*-ing, we can prevent or minimize the harm of these changes.

Stages of Addiction

The psychiatric community is moving away from using the word "addiction" because it can be seen as stigmatizing to call a person an "addict." For clarity, I am using the term "addiction" as a process, not in a pejorative or stigmatizing manner.

Addictions are usually defined in four stages:[525]

1. **Positive reward:** We feel a rush, an intoxication, a positive experience from the substance. This may move us toward binge-using the substance as our brain begins to associate the positive feelings with using the substance. We want to keep experiencing the "high." This is mediated by multiple areas of the brain, including the dopamine pathways in the "pleasure center." As you may remember from previous chapters, the dopamine pathways are also important in learning, motivation, concentration, sleep, and mood.

2. **Negative reward:** After some time, the "high" feeling turns into a "low" with feelings of irritability, dysphoria (dissatisfaction), and withdrawal. Our brain begins to associate the "low" feelings with *not* using the drug.

3. **Preoccupation:** Our brain drives us to seek substances to avoid the negative feelings of withdrawal. At this point, we can begin to lose control over our consumption of substances.

4. **Anticipation:** We seek out the substance to regulate our mood. Our focus becomes how we're going to obtain it and how we're going to feel once we've consumed it. This can become more powerful than the actual use of the substance itself.

Spectrum of Substance Use

In Figure 15.1, the spectrum of substance use is described as a range from abstinence to dangerous.[526] As you see in the figure, the use of some substances never moves past the non-problematic phase for most people—caffeine, which is technically considered a substance, is one such example. Caffeine also has recommended daily limits set by federal agencies that automatically fall at the non-problematic or below stage for many of us.

However, many substances, such as alcohol, can quickly become harmful and dangerous after use, especially in those of us with genetic factors putting them at greater risk of addiction. Indeed, for many of us, with or without the addictive gene or epigenetic changes, alcohol can become dangerous very quickly if misused.

FIGURE 15.1 FROM ABSTINENCE TO DANGEROUS USE OF SUBSTANCES [526]

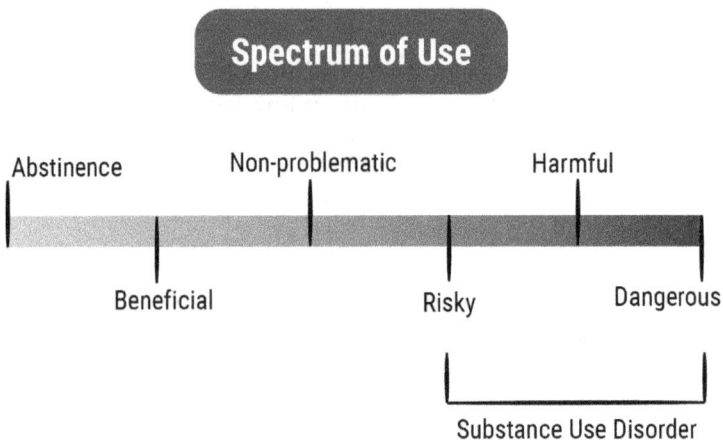

Spectrum of Use

Abstinence · Non-problematic · Harmful

Beneficial · Risky · Dangerous

Substance Use Disorder

At-risk drinking has been defined as more than five drinks a day by a male and more than four a day for a female. Assessments can also be done to help us understand if the substance use is problematic.[527] The CAGE Assessment is one such assessment that can help decide if someone falls into the "risky" or unhealthy area of substance use.

CAGE Assessment:[528]

1. Have you felt the need to **cut** down on your drinking or drug use?
2. Do you feel **annoyed** about people complaining about your drinking or drug use?
3. Do you ever feel **guilty** about your drinking or drug use?
4. Do you ever drink or use drugs as an **eye-opener** in the morning to relieve the shakes?

If you answer yes to one or more of these questions, maybe the time is now to assess how you can take control of your substance use. Take an inventory of potential blocks you have and *Restack* them using the tools we have discussed so far in the book. Consider what steps you can take to overcome these barriers. We've got this!

Looking at Substance Use Through the Pillars of Lifestyle Psychiatry

Lifestyle psychiatry and its pillars provide a solid organizational structure for thinking about substance use disorders. In this book, we have focused on multiple aspects of health, both mental and physical, and substance use transcends and overlaps many of these constructs. In the following section, we're going to drill down on the bidirectionality between substance use and these individual pillars. This section will be organized based on the more significant pillars for people struggling with substance use disorders, from most to least important in my clinical experience.

Sleep and Substance Use

Often, the first symptom seen in patients who subsequently develop substance use disorders is poor sleep, which we discussed in detail in Chapter 11. Specifically, for substance use disorders, poor sleep leads to changes in neuronal excitability and gene expression, among other brain changes.[529] This can predispose the sleep-deprived person to overconsume ultra-processed foods and often increases impulsivity during the day.

Substance abuse affects the architecture of sleep, with the duration and quality of the sleep, as well as the REM phase of sleep becoming impaired.[530] This can lead to decreased restful sleep overall, resulting in irritability and headaches.

The prevalence of sleep disorders in those misusing substances is astounding, with research showing between 36% to 91% of adults and about one-third of adolescents being affected.[531] As stated above, the relationship between sleep and substance use is bidirectional.[532] In fact, poor sleep is highly correlated with relapse.[533] The best-studied interventions include a specific type of therapy for insomnia called cognitive behavioral therapy-insomnia (CBT-I),[534] which was discussed in the sleep chapter and a self-help version is outlined in Rx 13.1 "Practicing Positive Cognitive Restructuring."

Connectedness and Substance Use

There's a good reason organizations like Alcoholics Anonymous (AA) use meetings to help people maintain sobriety.

Connectedness is exceedingly important for initiating abstinence and maintaining sobriety. A caring and supportive relationship with a healthcare clinician, loved one, sibling, or other family members can greatly assist an individual grappling with the shame and guilt often associated with substance use.[535]

Most individuals with substance use disorder have few social connections and experience higher rates of loneliness.[536] These individuals also often need to change their social network if it primarily includes others who are struggling in a similar vein.[537] Sometimes, improved social connection is not immediately possible while trying to find help. Therefore, other aspects of connectedness, which we discussed in Chapter 14, can be life-changing, including connecting with a higher power, finding a renewed purpose and meaning for existence, and engaging in a community, such as within a religious institution. Whatever leads us to removing the secrecy often associated with unhealthy substance use, and building trust with others is a step in the right direction.[538] We just need to take one step at a time.

Physical Activity and Substance Use

Increasing our physical activity and movement is important in combating substance use.[539] Exercise can improve depressive symptoms and ease anxiety and withdrawal symptoms.[540] These improvements were noted to be related to dopaminergic modification and BDNF,[541,542] which were described in Chapters 2 and 12. Physical activity also increases the release of serotonin from the raphe nuclei, which is another potential neurotrophic growth factor. It has also been shown that regular physical activity improves sleep quality, which leads to further reductions in substance use.

This interrelatedness between physical activity, sleep, and substance use is one example of how the concepts we presented in different chapters in this book are all parts of a whole. Indeed, lifestyle improvements and releasing our blocks in one area of our lives can translate to other areas.

Nutrition and Substance Use

Healthy intake of nutrients is a known problem for those struggling with substance use. Neglecting proper nutrition can lead to damage to the brain and digestive organs, like the intestines and liver. Research has found associations between substance use disorder and inadequate food intake, decreased fiber consumption, and poor absorption of nutrients, especially the B vitamins, iron, and magnesium.[543,544] The likelihood of eating ultra-high processed foods and struggling with food insecurity and malnutrition is higher in populations with substance use disorders.[545] The good news is due to the importance of the brain-gut microbiota system, eating more healthy foods can consequently be neuroprotective for those struggling with substance abuse.[546] The gut microbiota helps produce necessary components for brain health that may be depleted during substance use, such as short-chain fatty acids. Fiber and whole food, plant-based diets can have a tremendous impact on our overall health. The pillars of lifestyle psychiatry are interconnected, so when we address one, we may be addressing another. This is super amplified *Restack*-ing!

Stress and Substance Use

Stress reduction through mindfulness is helpful for everything—I know, this has been stated multiple times throughout this book—including struggles with substance use. Not being able to tolerate stress is a potential pathway for how those struggling with addiction can lose control. For this reason, mindfulness not only helps improve the anxiety associated with substance misuse but also the impulsivity to reach for the substance during times of stress.[547]

The mechanisms by which mindfulness treatments are helpful have been connected to reward processing and self-regulation in the brain, as described in Chapter 2. While the brain pathways are complex, the concepts are a bit easier. If you struggle in using them, maybe connect back to your "Why?" through Rx 9.2 "Developing Your 'Why?'" and by reviewing Rx 9.3 "Questions to Assess Your Cognitive Readiness for Change." These self-help techniques are often dismissed as "too simple" but are effective when done consistently over time.

What It Looks Like to Manage Substance Use Well

While our brains easily adapt to the changes the substances bring, they can also adapt to treatments once we stop using the substances. To effectively treat an addiction, we have to engage in healthy behaviors and activities that help the brain reshape. This process takes longer than developing the addictive behaviors, and it can get frustrating if one does not feel the immediate results.

Addiction is not only a behavioral problem but an emotional one as well. We already discussed in previous chapters some common emotional obstacles to behavior change. Two very useful techniques include mindfulness practices and root cause analysis. Let me describe them using the following case.

A Case of Pain Medication Misuse

Dawn is a 46-year-old patient who came in with an addiction to prescription pain medications. She had three children and was functioning well at work. She reported needing more and more pain meds to continue to maintain the state of numbness she was craving. During the first year of treatment, we didn't talk at all about stopping the pain meds. The conversation, rather, was about understanding what feelings Dawn was trying to avoid and going back to the *root cause* of those feelings, exploring how they started.

Over time, Dawn began to identify the root causes of her current addiction. She came to understand she hadn't processed the pain from being physically assaulted when she was 25 years old. She reflected on her history and noted that as her children were getting older, she didn't enjoy spending time with them. She became more and more obsessive and concerned about her physical safety, even without any apparent reason.

She began misusing prescription pain meds about five years before seeking treatment and found that as long as she was taking the meds, her obsessions moderated, and she wasn't as concerned for her physical safety.

As we used *mindfulness* techniques, such as breath work, visualizations, and music therapy, to help her calm herself, she was able to tolerate her feelings for the first time in many years. She spontaneously began the process of reframing the past and feeling stronger. She saw the pain meds as a crutch she no longer needed. During that process, helping her reengage with her kids and viewing that as a pleasurable interaction instead of something to avoid was essential in her recovery. By not immediately focusing on her addiction, we were able to empower her and over time, help her rediscover joy in her life.

First Steps Toward Treatment

Before you can have lasting change, you have to know your "Why?" Our whys are often connected to our inner purpose and meaning making that we talked about in Chapter 14.

Motivation to stop unhealthy substance use is a big hurdle many of us struggle with. One of the tools clinicians often employ is motivational interviewing, which is an opportunity for clinicians to partner with their patients. Obviously, not all of us are ready to quit misusing substances the first time they become a problem. As described before, Rx 9.1 "Developing Your 'Why?'" is a self-help adaptation of motivational interviewing techniques that may be useful for addressing unhealthy substance use.

The process of recovery is not a straight line. We will often progress and then face setbacks. Sometimes, even thinking about the plan you want to implement is the best you're going to be able to do in a day, and that is good enough. Let's stop the shame of saying to ourselves, "I didn't do what I wanted to do today." Instead, let's embrace the success of whatever movement we were able to make toward our goals, no matter how small it may seem. To borrow a sports cliché, winning ugly is still a win.

A Case of Alcohol Use Disorder

Stella is a 59-year-old software engineer at a tech startup and she said drinking is a part of the culture at work. She also has type 2 diabetes and had been noticing worsening blood sugar control over the last three months. Sometimes, she didn't even want to check her blood sugars because she knew how high they'd be. When she initially began seeing me, she was worried she might need to have a limb amputated, just like one of her relatives with diabetes recently had.

About three nights each week, Stella went out with friends and had three drinks each night. On the weekends, she had about five to six drinks a day. "Yeah, we sit out by the pool when it's warm, and I drink beers throughout the day." In total, she consumed over 20 drinks a week. At times, she had received comments from friends that she should cut back on her drinking. She was single at the time and wanted to get into a relationship, but her drinking led her to not remember many of her evenings.

Stella had tried to decrease her alcohol intake before, but after four days, she would get shaky and anxious and go back to drinking. She believed if she could get her sugars under control, then the other issues would sort themselves out. She had also gained 30 pounds in the last two years and noted feeling tired a lot. Her blood pressure was high, and liver enzymes were elevated on her labs.

Even with these kinds of lab results pointing to health problems from unhealthy substance use, the answer isn't always to immediately have Stella quit. First, she needed to be sufficiently *motivated* to quit. Stella and I discussed the option of quitting by giving her an easier first step of harm reduction through simply decreasing consumption. We explored the benefits of quitting versus decreasing alcohol use so she had the necessary information to make a decision. Even though some individuals with alcohol use disorder might be able to quit cold turkey, this can be very difficult for most. Instead, decreasing alcohol intake may be the more palatable first step. This process of giving Stella a choice allowed her *agency* over her healthcare decisions. Stella should be the one choosing what interventions she wanted to use.

Stella told me she was "sick and tired of feeling sick and tired." She opted to quit alcohol entirely, for a month, to see how it went. I involved her primary care physician and discussed possible withdrawal symptoms, some of which could be life-threatening, though one of the biggest challenges in working with Stella was her tech startup job did not provide health insurance. This barrier exists with many of my patients who, like her, are under-resourced and adds yet another challenge for those struggling with substance use disorders.

In our conversation about ways to still socialize and not drink, we had a good discussion outlining her options. She felt upbeat and excited about exploring mocktails (nonalcoholic mixed drinks). We also talked about the sugar content in mocktails and the importance of moderation. I encouraged her to try sparkling water with a wedge of lime as an alternative to avoid the high sugar content, especially given her diabetes. We continued to discuss her making new friends outside of the bar scene, so she would have options for other social outlets.

During her sessions with me, Stella reflected and said she did have a few work friends who don't drink and maybe she could spend more time with them. Over the next few months, Stella realized going to bars wasn't working for her as she had started drinking again. When she was at a bar, she felt pressured by people buying her drinks and became tempted to take shots when offered. She was initially embarrassed and hesitated to tell me that she went back to drinking. However, she found comfort in the gains she had made and was motivated to rework her plan.

She found joy in hanging out with the girlfriends from the Zumba class she recently joined. Also, she became closer friends with a few people in a diabetes education program. While she missed her old drinking buddies, and though she was still building her relationship with her new friends, she felt confident about being able to develop relationships outside of the bar. Stella's liver tests started trending to normal. She made plans to take salsa classes, with an eye toward entering a competition in the following year.

Stella's story highlights the slow and steady progress many of us ought to aim for when we are dealing with substance use. Her relapse was a "bump in the road," but she was able to reflect on it and not be deterred. Ultimately, it served as a motivation for her to push forward. While happy with her budding relationships, she never anticipated how many changes she would have to make in her social life. Stella showed tremendous courage, insight, and strength as she moved forward.

When we are first confronted with a pattern of our behaviors we want to change, the road forward often seems daunting. But assembling the right tools and systematically creating a structure that allows us to move forward incrementally—while also powering through some bumps along the way—can remove our barriers. Some of us may take a more linear path, while others may indeed need multiple tries to succeed. Just approach each new attempt with kindness and compassion toward yourself.

Other Types of Addictions

While addiction to substances is well-known and heavily researched, the emerging research about addiction is exploding! Connecting brain science research to other addictive behaviors will move the needle forward in what we know are already significant societal problems. Things like addiction to eating sugar? Sex and porn addiction? Gambling? Internet? Shopping? Gaming? Work? Exercise? All these addictions deserve consideration, and similar techniques to what I've described in this chapter can be employed to aid those of us struggling with these addictions. Let's look at a few of the largest concerns on this list to round out this chapter: sugar, social media, gaming, gambling, and pornography addiction.

Sugar Addiction

While foods with high refined and processed sugar content can become very addictive, many patients wonder about fruits. Are the sugars in fruits the same?

Fruits are healthy, and recent data shows that whole fruits consumed by those with type 2 diabetes can have protective and helpful effects in reversing the condition. Please consult your physician beforehand, though, if you have type 2 diabetes because not everyone responds the same way.[548] Fruit sugars have the beneficial fiber connected with them, which helps digest and regulate insulin. However, once the fiber is removed from the fruit by processing, certain receptors in the dopamine system can become altered, which can cause a change in mood.[549] If refined and processed sugar is eaten chronically, the receptor sensitivity to addictive substances changes, which is linked to the development of substance use disorders.

Social Media Addiction

Many researchers have noticed that since COVID-19, over 50% of people feel the effects of loneliness.[550,551] At the same time, we have also seen a trend of increased substance use, as well as increased use of social media and the Internet.[552,553] Many social media sites are designed to target the dopamine reward centers in our brain. With loneliness as a pervasive state for many people, it's no wonder that scrolling on our phones or increased time spent in front of the computer screen have become our companions—like an always accessible "friend."

Limiting screen time is a common recommendation by pediatricians and child psychiatrists. Indeed, too much screen time in infants and young children may disrupt normal brain development. Among young children, we've observed an explosive increase in ADHD and anxiety. Though the causes of this increase have yet to be worked out, it's hard not to wonder how much is related to these significant changes in what new generations of children are exposed to early on.

Gaming Addiction

Gaming addiction also follows a similar path to addictive substance use in our neuronal circuitry. Most of us would agree that playing games on or browsing the Internet can be healthy in moderation—even though sometimes that quick scroll may turn into hours.[554] Unfortunately, for many of us, the same loss of control, such as that occurring in the anticipation and preoccupation stages of addiction, may occur when we engage in these activities.

Gambling Addiction

Gambling addiction has expanded significantly with the invention of the internet. While initially categorized as an impulse control disorder, gambling has been recently reclassified as an addiction. Historically, less than 2% of the population was considered to be struggling with out of control gambling. With the internet, online gambling has been found to be exponentially growing, with wagering accounting for half of the online gambling market across the world. With high-speed internet, there is an increase in betting on fantasy sport leagues and sporting outcomes.[555] The other half includes casino games, poker, and bingo. The risk for vulnerable populations such as older adults and adolescents takes on new meaning with the increased availability of websites on the internet. The brain regions implicated include the ventromedial prefrontal cortex and the amygdala that are important in making everyday decisions and choices.[556] Dopamine dysregulation is also considered as a potential cause for gambling addiction. As with any hobby, many would categorize gambling as harmless in moderation, but when we lose control, it can cause potentially unfathomable disruptions in all areas of our lives. Many people frequently use substances, like alcohol, during periods of gambling to either heighten the thrill or cope with the losses.

Pornography Addiction

Online porn addiction shares similar mechanisms of actions as other addictions and may be a subclassification of sex addictions.[557] While hypersexual disorder may be seen in about 5% of the population, online pornography addiction is considered much more prevalent.[558] Data supports that many users of internet porn do not think they have a problem or an addiction.[558] With any viewing of online pornography, there is a change in sexual satisfaction with some studies suggesting that consumers of online experienced diminished pleasure during real-life sexual encounters.[558] Other studies have shown increased dissatisfaction with performance, partners, and their own bodies.[559] Brain changes include studies showing impaired responses to stress, desensitization of pleasure requiring more and more stimulation for the same level of arousal, and changes in the amygdala similar to what's seen in extraordinary stress.[560] For many, the increased use of pornography leads to disrupted family life and worsening substance use.

Conclusion

Something "normal" for society could be unraveling for many of us. Our modern culture and social lives often normalize drinking and other substance use. Often, people can manage their lives without letting these substances take over or cause negative health consequences. But this chapter is about empowering those who have lost control, or are at risk of losing control, of their substance use to the point where it is hurting them and their loved ones. Our conversation here is about each person's need to improve their overall health and quality of life. Substance use treatment is not about judgment, but instead about supporting a person making a decision to reel in a behavior they don't like or wanting to make a positive change in their life. This is the most important step.

Chapter 16: Beyond Self-Help

Let's honor what makes us unique and human. We are inherently different, so we need individualized approaches to treatment.

One of my goals for writing this book was to impart knowledge through my lived experiences and my 30-plus years as a psychiatrist. Through my own personal growth, I have changed dramatically in these last few decades, and I suspect many readers find this true in their lives as well. Growth often does not follow a direct or sequential path. A tool that may not be a good fit for you now may be the gold you're looking for later in life.

The lifestyle psychiatry concepts we discussed are new and employ a different lens for looking at illnesses. Making this research available to a general audience is why I felt compelled to write *Restack*. But are the solutions I present in this book the ultimate answers for 100% of people, at every stage of their life? No. An absolute resounding no.

Sometimes, we might need other interventions beyond self-help. In the previous chapters, I have written about times when I was in psychotherapy, and it was exceedingly helpful. However, not all psychotherapies are the same. In my late thirties, I engaged in cognitive behavioral therapy (CBT). When my trauma created internal blocks, I engaged in eye movement desensitization and reprocessing (EMDR) therapy and a novel version called accelerated resolution therapy (ART). Psychodynamic psychotherapy helped me progress at other times, and in my early 30s, I was in psychoanalytic treatment. All these treatments were reparative and beneficial, but at different points in my life.

I wish I could guide each individual reader in figuring out what may be helpful for them at any given point in their lives. But as *just an author*, I have to live with the fact that I cannot. What I can do is lay out the information, with the intention of providing education, so you can make the best decision for you. Please do consider a comprehensive psychiatric evaluation if you are struggling to make the progress you need to by yourself.

I don't believe this can be stated often enough: We are all different, and we necessarily *need* to have an individualized approach to our treatment.

Formal Psychological and Psychiatric Help

The highest form of "self-help" is knowing when you need *more* than self-help.

Knowing when to seek formal treatment versus relying on self-help can profoundly impact your well-being and ability to effectively address the challenges and obstacles in your life. It's crucial to recognize that seeking formal help does not indicate weakness or failure. Rather, it shows a proactive strategy to tackle complex issues and prioritize your needs— seeking the right help for yourself is the ultimate act of self-love. Combining self-help resources with professional support whenever needed can establish a comprehensive approach to personal growth and well-being.

It's advisable to seek formal treatment if you face severe mental health concerns such as severe anxiety, depression, and suicidal thoughts. In the U.S., we have a dedicated 24-hour suicide and crisis lifeline: 988.

Severe trauma and grief can strain our coping mechanisms, and professional support can provide guidance and healing during difficult times. Long-standing personal or interpersonal challenges, substance use disorders, persistent relationship conflicts, learning differences, and communication stalemates are all situations where a professional can offer valuable insights, strategies, and structured interventions to effectively address underlying issues.

Broadly, formal help can be divided into therapy, including psychotherapy and other forms, medication, coaching, and peer support groups. Outside of these major categories, more restrictive options are available for more severe issues, such as inpatient treatment, intensive outpatient programs, residential treatment, and rehabilitation centers.

Rest assured, going to a professional doesn't mean you can't continue the self-help path outlined in this book. In fact, they can complement each other quite well. There are also alternative options outside of mainstream medicine you can explore.

Types of Interventions Available in Medicine

I am a psychiatrist working in conventional medicine, which means I view diseases through a particular lens. Please see Table 16.1 for a breakdown of different specialty areas in medicine.[561-568]

While this book did not address functional medicine, complementary and alternative medicine (CAM), and other unconventional approaches to care in detail, I believe they may be useful for some people. Indeed, I've also dabbled and used these treatments for myself at times. While I do not provide any of these nonconventional medicine treatments for my patients, I recognize their potential benefits. These non-conventional treatments are just not within the realm of conventional medicine and, therefore, not considered lifestyle psychiatry and/or lifestyle medicine.

Why am I focusing on the differences between these commonly available treatment modalities? Because these distinctions are pivotal for us to understand so we can choose wisely and make informed decisions about our health. For instance, CAM uses a fundamentally different approach to conceptualizing organs and disease states compared to conventional medicine. In conventional medicine, clinicians talk about kidney disease or liver disease, whereas in CAM they may instead focus on energy states and the meridian system of the body. Some of the approaches used in

CAM include acupuncture, Ayurvedic medicine, homeopathic medicine, reiki, and energy healing.

Table 16.1 Different Seemingly Overlapping Areas of Specialty Medicine[561]			
Specialty Area	Definition	Areas of Emphasis	Evidence-based?
Conventional medicine[562]	Routine, mainstream allopathic medicine that is rigorously focused on evidence-based practices and typically emphasizes symptom management or amelioration.	• Medication • Surgery • Symptoms	Yes
Lifestyle medicine[563, 564]	An active evidence-based management process that utilizes the same approach to understand the psychopathology and diagnosis of diseases as conventional medicine but differs in that lifestyle medicine focuses on preventing and reversing disease for individuals.	• Diet and eating • Physical activity • Sleep • Relationships • Substance use risk reduction • Stress management	Yes
Integrative medicine[565]	An approach that emphasizes all available treatment modalities, including conventional and alternative.	• Lifestyle medicine can be a core aspect • Healing-oriented • Emphasizes mind-body-spirit intersection	Sometimes
Functional medicine[566]	A model that attends to and treats the dynamic process that results in dysfunction or disease, rather than the disease itself.	• Focused on function, not pathology • Personalized care based on biochemical individuality	Sometimes

Table 16.1 Different Seemingly Overlapping Areas of Specialty Medicine (continued)			
Preventative medicine	Specialty area of practice that focuses on health promotion of individuals as well as communities.	• Overlaps with public health • Three subspecialties include (1) public health and general preventive medicine, (2) occupational medicine, and (3) aerospace medicine	Yes
Complementary and alternative medicine (CAM)	Wide range of preventative and therapeutic modalities, which may not be evidence-based, and may be influenced by providers' own values and philosophies.	• Examples include acupuncture, chiropractic care, and reiki	Rarely

Adopting Emerging Research into Mainstream Medicine

In conventional medicine, for an intervention to be adopted as mainstream, it is required to undergo rigorous research, including randomized control trials and replication of the results in future studies. This standard can be problematic for some lifestyle studies as randomization isn't always possible or ethical. Many interventions have not made it to mainstream medicine, and I would classify them as emerging interventions or soon-to-be mainstream conventional medicine. I have found these treatments beneficial for some of my patients. Table 16.2 includes some of these emerging treatments, which can be used for overall wellness in the primordial prevention stage we described in Chapter 7: Burnout, or for disease treatment and reversal.

Treatments for Mental Health Disorders

Psychotherapies can be easily classified into two major types of therapies: those addressing the here-and-now and those looking into a patient's past and how it informs current behaviors and feelings. Therapies that address the here-and-now tend to be used for a shorter duration and are suitable for people whose symptoms are not deeply rooted in long-standing patterns developed over many years. Sometimes, we may start with these surface-level therapies and then realize we may need to go deeper. When I assess patients, that's the conversation we have. Some people immediately opt to begin the deeper work of untangling past patterns or experiences, while others choose to sit with the current symptoms and attempt something like CBT. Though this book is not meant to go into detail about all the available mental health interventions, I have included a summary of some therapies for your consideration in Table 16.2.

It's important to acknowledge that within each category, numerous specific therapeutic models and techniques may be available. Additionally, some therapists may integrate multiple approaches to create a tailored treatment plan for their patients. The choice of psychotherapy depends on the individual's unique circumstances, preferences, and therapeutic goals. As people differ in their experiences, personalities, and challenges, therapeutic interventions must be varied and flexible to address individual needs effectively. Each approach offers a distinct perspective on human behavior, emotions, and cognitive processes, allowing therapists to tailor their interventions based on the patient's specific condition and preferences.

Table 16.2 Types of Therapies for Mental Health Disorders

Type of Treatment	Overview
Acceptance and Commitment Therapy (ACT)	ACT is a newer intervention that uses acceptance, mindfulness, and commitment behavior change strategies, with the goal of increasing psychological flexibility. ACT is not limited by time, and the patient plays a larger role in laying out their treatment (compared to CBT).
Animal-assisted Therapy	Animal-assisted therapy can be implemented individually or in groups. This therapy improves connectedness through improvements in physical, social, emotional, and cognitive functioning.
Cognitive Behavioral Therapy (CBT)	CBT focuses on thoughts, patterns, and behaviors and how they influence each other. CBT encourages the patient to recognize their negative thoughts and develop techniques to modify thought patterns and behaviors. CBT is a clinician-led, time-limited therapy.
Dialectical Behavior Therapy (DBT)	DBT emphasizes regulating emotions, learning to accept painful situations, and encouraging mindfulness. DBT stresses regulating harmful and destructive behavioral patterns. DBT is a clinician-led, time-limited therapy.
Eclectic Approaches	This approach combines techniques from various other types of therapies, in order to flexibly adjust based on the needs of the patient. This is commonly practiced by many therapists.
Exposure Therapy	This therapy creates an environment to help individuals gradually confront the fear and avoidance related to certain activities or situations. It is commonly used in anxiety disorders, like fear of flying or fear of spiders. This therapy needs to be carefully used, as it has the potential to cause more harm than good in people with significant trauma, such as posttraumatic stress disorder.
Eye movement desensitization and reprocessing (EMDR)	EMDR is an eye movement structured therapy to reduce the vivid emotions and distress associated with traumatic memories. It can be used in certain situations, such as military combat, physical assault, and car accidents.
Accelerated resolution therapy (ART)	ART is a newer form of eye movement therapy that expands on EMDR techniques. ART adds a component of narrative imagery to replace disturbing traumatic images with pleasant ones.

Both EMDR and ART are time-limited therapies, with many experiencing relief within one to five sessions. |

Table 16.2 Types of Therapies for Mental Health Disorders (continued)

Family and Couples therapy	This clinician-led therapy works with families or couples with the aim to enhance communication, identify and manage conflicts, build stronger relationships, and overall improve the functioning of the family or couple.
Group therapy	A therapist-led group of individuals with a similar shared experience meets at regular times (in person or virtually). The aim is to provide support, foster connectedness, and learn from each other.
Humanistic therapies	These modalities focus on the patient's search for meaning and purpose in their lives. The therapy is more positively focused on growth and self-actualization. Examples include Gestalt Therapy, logotherapy, narrative therapy, and patient-centered therapy. Many therapists include a humanistic approach to their practice.
Hypnosis	Hypnosis is usually performed with a clinician by creating a changed state of awareness, with decreased awareness of the outside. This allows the patient to be more susceptible to suggestions.
Self-hypnosis	Self-hypnosis is a commonly used modality that offers benefits to many. One commonly used technique is listening to subliminal self-help messages.
Interpersonal Therapy (IPT)	IPT focuses on current problems, specifically in relationships, without delving into childhood issues. The aim is to improve interpersonal relationships that contribute to distress and emotional conflicts.
Mindfulness-based Therapies	These therapies use specific mindfulness practices to improve awareness and reduce stress. They can be clinician-led or practiced alone in a self-help manner. Examples include Mindfulness-Based Stress Reduction (MBSR) and Mindfulness-Based Cognitive Therapy (MBCT).
Psychoanalysis	Psychoanalysis is a treatment that involves bringing aspects of ourselves that we are not aware of (unconscious) to our awareness (conscious). This creates insight into our childhood, current relationships, emotional responses, and choices that we make. Psychoanalysis is not for everyone, as it can be costly and time-consuming. Many have benefited over the decades by removing blocks standing in the way of reaching one's potential and happiness.

Table 16.2 Types of Therapies for Mental Health Disorders (continued)	
Psychodynamic Psychotherapy (also called Insight-oriented Psychotherapy)	This therapy focuses on exploring unconscious aspects (blocks) of our lives, including thoughts, feelings, and past experiences. It delves into the root causes of emotional difficulties, with an emphasis on growth and healing. This is clinician-led and not limited by time.
Red Light Therapy (also called Photobiomodulation)	Hundreds of research papers have shown the benefits of red light therapy for multiple illnesses and overall rejuvenation. Athletes are using red light therapy to assist with muscle recovery, and instruments exist that are used by almost every professional sports group in the US. This is different from bright light therapy (used for mood disorders).
Supportive Psychotherapy	This approach uses techniques from other types of therapies, such as active listening and emotional support, with the aim of building the patient's confidence and self-esteem. This is clinician-led and not limited by time.
Trauma-informed Therapy	Therapy is provided by a clinician who, first and foremost, is sensitive to the complex effects of trauma and how those inform coping. The therapist continues the awareness of trauma in every aspect of the treatment. The treatment may be any of the other therapies listed in this table.

Coaching

Coaching can be a potent tool in improving our confidence and achieving our goals.

Coaching is a dynamic and transformative process offering numerous benefits to individuals seeking personal and professional growth. One of the primary advantages of coaching is the opportunity to gain clarity and focus on specific goals. Coaches work closely with people to help them identify their aspirations, values, and ambitions, assisting them in articulating clear and achievable objectives. By setting well-defined goals, clients can create a roadmap for success and stay motivated to take actionable steps toward their desired outcomes. Coaches serve as supportive partners who hold clients accountable for their commitments and progress. Regular check-ins and feedback from the coach keep clients on track and encourage them to take responsibility for their actions. This accountability fosters discipline, commitment, and ultimately greater success for clients.

A word of caution is to make sure you receive a professional comprehensive evaluation before engaging in coaching. While coaching can be effective for addressing specific goals and challenges, it is necessarily narrow and often doesn't delve into our overall psychological needs. Coaching is an approach regularly used by lifestyle medicine clinicians who can perform a comprehensive evaluation or refer you to a mental health provider.

We will present the case of Anna, who was referred to a coach for her struggles with her weight, to highlight a coaching approach. Coaches tend to employ motivational interviewing techniques, which we discussed in Chapter 9: *Restack* Model of Change, when working with their clients.

A Case of Coaching

When Anna, a 26-year-old woman, wanted to lose 40 pounds, her coach encouraged her to break down her goals into chunks that were more attainable over short periods of time. Rather than fixating on weight, Anna's coach emphasized manageable behavior change with a high likelihood of success. Anna identified her "why" as wanting to feel more comfortable dancing at her cousin's wedding, which was coming up in six months, and to feel overall more confident about her body.

Anna's initial goals were to work out twice a week, with weights, at 7 am on Tuesday and Friday for 45 minutes, followed by a 10-minute cardio sprint. She assessed her potential for success in completing these goals as a 9 out of 10. Anna and her coach continued to meet regularly to assess her progress and refine her goals accordingly. If Anna didn't meet a goal over time, it would evolve to a new goal she felt more confident she could achieve. If she felt she did not make progress on her goals, her coach assisted her in reframing the conversation and guiding her to identify a positive thought, feeling, or action around her goals. Thus, Anna was able to recognize the strides she had accomplished, even if she had not reached her previous goal.

As demonstrated in Anna's case, coaching can be a powerful tool to facilitate behavioral change. I've observed that many of my patients have derived benefit from working directly with coaches for a short period of time. However, in situations where my patient felt "stuck" or were not benefiting from coaching, I often recommended for them to consider formal psychotherapy or a peer support (self-help) group so they could meet others with similar goals.

The Power of Peer Support (Self-Help) Groups

Sometimes what we need is a peer to listen, understand, and support us— the metaphorical "village."

Peer support groups, also known as self-help groups or mutual support groups, are composed of individuals who share similar challenges or experiences. These individuals come together to provide emotional support, understanding, and practical guidance to one another. Unlike traditional therapy sessions led by professional therapists or counselors, peers typically lead peer support groups. Peers nurture a nonclinical and supportive environment where individuals can connect with others who have faced similar struggles. Also, unlike traditional therapy settings, peer support groups operate without hierarchical structures. All participants are equal members, thereby encouraging a greater sense of comfort in sharing and connecting with each other.

Peer support groups offer a sense of belonging and validation as participants realize they are not alone in their experiences. Sharing similar challenges cultivates an understanding and empathetic environment where participants can freely and openly express themselves. Peer support groups often serve to empower individuals to take an active role in their own recovery and growth. As they provide support to others, participants often find developing a sense of purpose with their contributions, enhancing their self-esteem and resilience.

Peer support groups can cover a wide range of topics and issues, catering to various needs and interests. These groups also provide considerable flexibility as they can take various formats, such as face-to-face in-person meetings and online forums. This ensures greater accessibility for individuals regardless of location or mobility.

Examples of community peer-led self-help groups include:

1. The twelve-step program groups:
    - Alcoholics Anonymous (AA)
    - Narcotics Anonymous (NA)
    - Overeaters Anonymous (OA)
    - Sex Addicts Anonymous (SAA)
    - Co-Dependents Anonymous (CoDA)
2. National Alliance on Mental Illness (aids those with mental illness and their families to find support within the community)
3. American Foundation for Suicide Prevention

Other Resources

Community mental health centers often offer sliding-scale fees or free counseling services to make treatment more accessible. Online resources, such as forums and apps, can provide valuable insights and peer support, especially for those with mobility challenges. Public health clinics might offer addiction-related services at reduced costs, while free helplines can connect individuals to trained counselors. Some universities and nonprofit organizations like religious institutions may also offer low-cost or no-cost counseling options. Utilizing self-help books and materials available at libraries can also offer strategies and guidance. While accessing professional treatment may pose financial challenges, identifying and taking advantage of available community resources and peer support can be crucial steps in our journeys toward recovery.

Path Forward

At any point in our lives, we are a summary statement of our lived experiences and genetics.

We have evolved along various trajectories to reach where we are today, and we will continue to evolve. Given this, certain interventions may work for certain people at certain times in their lives. What worked for you five years ago may not speak to you now because you're a different person, both biologically and in your life experiences. I hope this chapter has provided you with new tools to add to your toolbox as you navigate your journey of *Restack*-ing.

Professional help like medication and formal psychotherapy can be invaluable at times. Many of us have experimented with different types of therapy, coaching, and self-help books to guide us on our journeys. This chapter has offered an overview of the available theoretical frameworks or approaches, each with their own benefits. None of these approaches is one-size-fits-all—it depends on where we are in our journeys and what we currently need.

Chapter 17: With Gratitude and in Health

Let's honor our flaws, mistakes, and the experiences that have led us here.

So, this is the point where we step back and reflect on who we are, where we've been, and what we want to do to navigate our futures. In my life, it's taken me a long time to distill the insights I've shared in these chapters. I've made numerous blunders and spent countless hours in reflection. I've shared some of those slipups with you among these pages. But being honest and vulnerable is only part of the process of growth. By extending myself grace, compassion, and love, I've learned to focus on celebrating my wins—each day, every hour, every month, and every year. A mindset emphasizing positivity and putting the emotional and material roadblocks I've had into perspective (often with humor!) has been lifesaving for me.

Hopefully, in reading this book, you were able to identify some areas that spark excitement as you embrace the path of releasing your mental blocks and *Restack*-ing your potential. The Rx's in these chapters can be referred to time and time again and can be important to overcoming the emotional, cognitive, personality, and behavioral limitations you experience. We don't have control over many aspects of our existence. We can't choose our genetics or many of the factors in our environments, but we do possess the capacity to influence our own individual happiness. This can be achieved by actively choosing how we engage with and understand our lived experiences.

This begs us to contemplate the question: What is happiness? As explored in this book, I'm not talking about *just* hedonism, but also a sense of peace and a maximal potential for joy. Throughout history, every generation has sought to find better ways to engage with the world, with the overarching goal of discovering both our individual and collective happiness. I believe the concepts presented in this book have a place in the conversation. With recent generations questioning many aspects of how we have constructed our society—work-life balance, marriage, religion, wars, etc.—these existential questions, intertwined with our personal journeys, are pivotal in working toward optimal health.

We are actively questioning the nature of work, the status quo of the 9-to-5, and how that affects our mental health and well-being. We wonder if a five-day workweek is the way our society needs to work anymore. The Industrial Revolution dramatically changed our way of life and refined human tasks in the workplace. Are we, perhaps, at the precipice of another major shift? As a society, we have arrived at a place where we're questioning the overreliance on experts and wondering if they've caused us to veer in the wrong direction. In the same breath, we are questioning the value of institutional education and a four-year college degree. We're asking ourselves, "Do we need to learn in academic institutions as they currently are? Is there a better way?"

In this book, I am asking comparable questions, but about aspects of our lifestyle that have just started to become part of the mainstream conversation, namely our overreliance on ultra-processed foods and our sedentary habits. Are we ready to remove the mental blocks and external barriers holding many of us hostage in our suffering and preventing us from realizing our dreams? Though sometimes these are issues we are not ready to face or process within ourselves, they are crucial to address if we wish to progress toward achieving our full potential.

We have power over our lifestyle only to the degree our environment allows. Let me state it another way: If our external environment is toxic and fails to bring out the best of us, despite our efforts to improve, we can be limited in the power that a healthy lifestyle can afford us. With the anticipated growth of artificial intelligence and other world changes beyond our control, our external environment becomes nebulous. Many of us are worried about being replaced in our jobs by artificial intelligence and the current global tensions between countries. While these potential realities are beyond our control, on an individual level, we need to remain grounded and strive to function at the highest possible level we can.

Indeed, even if we cannot change our external environment, we can change how we view it and our mindset. That is, we can change our internal environment through the process of *Restack*-ing. Let's get back on the road of living a life of health and experiencing every ounce of joy possible in this human existence.

What has become abundantly clear to me in writing this book, and in living my life, is I don't know all the answers. I understand only some of the questions. And I experientially know what has worked for me and for my patients for the last 30-plus years.

I am so excited about the future of our new generation, with their curiosity and their rebellious questioning and distancing from cultural norms. They are unwilling to accept the status quo. It's refreshing and needed in the current state of our world. We each have the capacity to transform our own lives and harness the power of our brain in the process.

As this book comes to a close, let me end as I end all my emails, with grace and love toward myself, and toward you...

With gratitude and in health,

Gia Merlo

Epilogue

Now 60 years old, after having lived in New York, Philadelphia, Houston, and Louisiana, I've settled down in a home minutes away from my daughter and her family. Looking back at my journey, full of its sorrow, intense psychological work, joy, happiness, and so many memorable life-altering moments, I can't help but feel a pang of nostalgia. Many of us feel lucky if we've had one or two moments that define who we are, and we make life choices that speak to our soul and our character, but as I write this, I can count a dozen or more. I needed all those pivots in my life. And through the evolution and "growth spurts" I endured as an adult, I reconsolidated myself to a higher level of functioning. Indeed, *Restack* is my modus operandi.

I am at a place of peace internally and not struggling at the level I have in my life previously. I have a stable, loving relationship with myself and those around me. I tear up when I see love and joy being expressed. And I shed tears when I see the suffering of others. I enjoy these emotional connections without the overlay of trauma.

This is my fifth book. The first four academic books were to help me get to a place where I could write *Restack*. Sharing what I've learned in an open, vulnerable way is about removing the stigma and shame around mental suffering, removing the pretense that, though *externally* we may look well put together, we may be suffering inside. This effort is not only for sharing my story, but also hopefully to inspire others to face their mental blocks with courage and to develop a lifestyle that resonates with the deepest part of their soul.

We all have one life. How do we want to live it? Do we want to live it with chronic mental or physical diseases, or with health? This is the question we all have to ask ourselves. Let's collectively *Restack* what's not working and free ourselves. Let's embrace the four-letter word that is so hard for many of us to say, much less experience, for ourselves and for others: love.

I plan to slow down my life and live with more intention by taking up hobbies that have fallen by the wayside over the years, like practicing my violin, joining a community orchestra, taking dance classes, starting up tennis again, and maybe even learning how to play pickleball. I am freeing up space to enjoy and invest in myself. I have been delaying this for so long—I am the queen of delayed gratification. I have visions of taking day hikes in the forest, spending time loving family and friends, hanging out by the pool, and reading novels for pleasure. Of course, I'm going to continue to do what I've always enjoyed—including mentoring budding health professionals, volunteering in the community, teaching, seeing patients, and passionately working to move lifestyle psychiatry and lifestyle medicine forward in the collective conversation.

All the while, you will see me out and about, belly laughing daily and counting my blessings.

Acknowledgments

As a practicing psychiatrist for over 30 years, I have many people to thank. Always first and foremost I am grateful for the patients who have trusted me with their care. Your courage and vulnerability have fueled my own. My evolution as a human necessarily involves me thanking my family and my therapists over the years--though you may not have heard me say it clearly before--your missteps and imperfections have given me permission to own mine.

Professionally, I have received mentorship from many through the decades. I especially want to thank my friend and mentor Jim Rippe for his ongoing trust in me and embracing the importance of mental health in the field of lifestyle medicine. His faith in me allowed the two books, *Lifestyle Nursing* and *Lifestyle Psychiatry*, to see the light of day. Equally supportive have been the hundreds of colleagues, many whom I now call friends, in the American College of Lifestyle Medicine including staff members and other leaders. Saying thank you to them doesn't seem like enough, but I am so grateful.

Collaboration with Christopher P. Fagundes in publishing *Lifestyle Psychiatry* expanded my capacity to truly understand the latest research in behavioral medicine and how that informs lifestyle interventions. I would not have been able to consolidate and synthesize this knowledge into my own health and share it via this book without the internal process of editing the book. Thank you, Chris, and to all the contributing authors of *Lifestyle Psychiatry* for helping me in ways you may not even realize.

So many people have been a part of the journey of writing this book. I especially want to thank those who supported me in the early stages, many of whom served as beta readers and are dear friends, including Liana Abascal, Josie Bidwell, Deborah Chielli, Beth Frates, Robert Gluck, Meagan Grega, Amy Hanus, Thomas Harter, Mary Horton,

Erika Kawamura, Eric Koester, Karen Laing, Lianna Levine Reisner, Monisha Lewis, Liana Lianov, Megan Marumoto, Sapna Moudgil-Shah, Ariyaneh Nikbin, Hugo Ortega, Laurie Robinson, Ali Saad, Janine Santora, Urvi Shah, Elizabeth Simkus, Susan Spell, Cody Stubbe, Steve Sugden, Carolyn Sweetapple, Karen Theesen, Michelle Tollefson, Cheryl True, Alyssa Vela, and Wendi Waits.

While this book is self-published, I created a team of phenomenal human beings who helped me along the way, including Steve Sugden, Monisha Lewis, Deborah Chielli, Megan Marumoto, Thomas Harter, Ali Saad, and Karen Laing who provided feedback for earlier chapters. Thank you to Aime Sund for your excellent copy editing, going above and beyond the call of duty.

Monisha Lewis, Wayne Lewis, and Torin Lewis have given me hope for the next generation, and for this, I am overjoyed. I especially want to thank Monisha Lewis and Steve Sugden, who patiently read the first book draft. Monisha (as my family) and Steve (as my work colleague working together to advance the lifestyle psychiatry movement) gave me permission to publish this book, and they both promised they would not be embarrassed by the vulnerability and personal content contained herein. I am going to hold them to it. Also, a special note of thanks to Katharine Smith and Catherine Clarke for saving the day and getting this book to the finish line!

Last but not least, I want to express my gratitude to Ariyaneh Nikbin, M.D. who has stood by me in this book-writing journey, from the first incarnation in 2020 to the mad dash to write this book over the last few months, while she was in her fourth year of medical school (and now a new doctor). The conversations, concept development, and clarification, along with her editorial assistance, were indispensable in the creation of this book. And I can't wait to hear her stories of healing and how she moves our field and society forward as a future psychiatrist.

Thank you. All of you.

References:

To view the cited sources and references in the book, please go to the following: https://www.giamerlo.com/citations-for-restack.

Alternatively, please scan the QR code below with your phone camera:

www.ingramcontent.com/pod-product-compliance
Lightning Source LLC
Chambersburg PA
CBHW022043020426
42335CB00012B/518